Just One Bite

Just One Bite

A FOOD ALLERGY MOM'S
SEARCH FOR ANSWERS

Meghan Neri

To request permission, contact the publisher at:
publisher@innerpeacepress.com

ISBN: 978-1-958150-14-6
Just One Bite: A Food Allergy Mom's Search for Answers

First edition June 2023
Cover image by: Lauren Cole Imagery

Subjects
HEALTH & FITNESS / Allergies
SELF-HELP / Anxieties & Phobias
COOKING / Health & Healing / Allergy

Published by Inner Peace Press
Eau Claire, Wisconsin, USA
www.innerpeacepress.com

To Shea and Thomas, I love you with all my heart. I'm so proud of your compassion, your empathy, and your resiliency. Fly my babies, fly.

To Jay, I love you. How blessed I am to hold your hand every step of the way.

Table of Contents

Praise for
Just One Bite

"A heart-warming narrative about one family's journey of learning how to navigate life with life-threatening food allergies. You'll sympathize and learn from reading Meghan's family stories navigating family parties, school food policies, babysitters, food anxieties, and more. As a mother of a food allergic child myself, I could be found exclaiming, "So true!" and "I totally get this!" as I read."

~Francesca Rose, President of UFAN (Utah Food Allergy Network, a non-profit food allergy resource with a Medical Advisory Board. UFAN's mission is to provide outreach to the newly diagnosed and the community at large, offering support, promoting education, building awareness of the severity of food allergies and anaphylaxis, and advocating for positive change.

"A must read for a newly diagnosed food allergy parent! Meghan gives us a truly relatable inside look at the journey her family is on from a parent's perspective, navigating the tough terrain those of us with food allergy children face. Our family can relate to the feelings of anxiety, loneliness, and desires for education, inclusion, and empathy. If only we had a book like this to understand our new chapter of life that began the day our daughter was diagnosed with life-threatening food allergies."

~Lisa Heath, Co-Founder of Intentional Foods (IF) Cafe & Market Working together with her husband, Ned Heath, IF provides the community with allergy-friendly meals and fosters an inclusive dining experience.

"This memoir is an amazing resource for families and children with food allergies. As an educator and entertainer, I know how important it is to create a safe and inclusive environment for all children, regardless of their allergies. It's inspiring to hear personal stories that shed light on the challenges of living with food allergies and offer practical solutions and resources to help manage them. By sharing her family's story and including helpful resources, Meghan raises awareness about food allergies and provides a valuable tool for families and caregivers. I'm sure many will benefit from reading this book and discovering new ways to cope with food allergies."

~Kyle Dine, Musician and Allergy Educator performs highly-acclaimed educational school presentations he developed about food allergies to over 900 schools in North America. Kyle is also the CEO and Founder of Equal Eats, a diet-tech start-up offering dietary communication cards.

Disclaimer

What is my lane? Mom? Advocate? Educator? I'm a teacher turned "stay-at-home mom" who has learned a lot about food allergies over the years. I see gaps and I have ideas for increasing education and promoting awareness. I know I'm not an allergist or a doctor or a nurse. I don't mean to get myself confused with things that are medical. But, here's the thing... Allergists don't have time (with the exception of a few, like Dr. Michael Pistiner, who you will read about later). School nurses don't have time. Pediatricians don't have time. So whose responsibility is it to educate? There are great resources out there but I'm talking about person-to-person learning. Being able to ask questions in real time. After years of managing multiple life-threatening food allergies and being a support group leader, I've determined I want to be a Food Allergy Educator. My journey, my family's journey, has led me to this conclusion. I have created trainings. I have made sure everything I put together is available to the public from respected sources, most of which can also be found in the pages of this book. I take information and put it on a silver platter. I consider my lane to be part of the bridge between diagnosis and everyday life. This means educating anyone, whether they manage food allergies or not. I'm a mom, an advocate, and an educator.

Foreword

As a family therapist working with parents of food allergic children and teens, I've spent many hours exploring allergy parenting experiences – each one unique and very personal.

The reality is that living with life-threatening food allergy involves navigating uncertainty and unpredictability, both of which are common anxiety triggers. While parents are provided with evidence-based allergy management guidelines, each family navigates this guidance differently.

Parents of food allergic children travel through a complex parenting journey, tasked with navigating stressful intricacies on a daily basis. While focused on their child's safety, they also need to allow necessary childhood development tasks to occur at the same time. Needless to say, this can feel incredibly daunting!

Therefore, it should come as no surprise that parenting a child with a potentially life-threatening food allergy can be very emotional. Parents may toggle between periods of confidence and hesitancy, experiencing anxiety, fear, sadness, grief, trauma, anger, and even relief, especially if the food allergy diagnosis provided answers to a confusing set of symptoms. And parents aren't the only ones who are impacted, as a food allergy diagnosis can be an emotional journey for the entire family system.

With all of that said, it IS possible to live life to its fullest even with a potentially life-threatening food allergy! This book is a beautiful example of this, illustrating how developing a workable balance between allergy-related fear and courage positively impacts a family's quality of life.

Meghan's relatable experiences will emotionally validate parents of food allergic children, enabling them to feel understood and part of a growing community. Taking readers along on her own parenting journey, Meghan shares how she moved from disbelief to acceptance, allowing her to approach food allergy life with an empowered mindset and the ability to advocate, support, and educate others.

Additionally, this book shares creative ideas for handling common food allergy experiences, and provides a list of reputable resources that are sure to benefit families managing food allergies.

Simply put, if you're looking for a beacon of hope and examples of how to develop a path through the challenges of parenting a child with a potentially life-threatening food allergy, this is the book for you!

Tamara Hubbard, MA, LCPC

An allergy-informed Licensed Clinical Professional Counselor, Tamara regularly works with parents of children managing allergic diseases in her private practice. She's the founder and CEO of The Food Allergy Counselor, and is an allied health member of both the American Academy of Allergy, Asthma and Immunology, and the American College of Allergy, Asthma and Immunology. Additionally, she's an international presenter on allergy mental health-related topics.

Introduction

Food allergies aren't a choice. Not for a child, not for their parents, not for the family. When you learn your child has a food allergy you are inducted into a club you never asked to join.

Jay and I often hear, "So one of you must have food allergies." Nope. We don't. We were novices in this foreign landscape. Thrown into the deep end. I think people hear about life with food allergies and can't imagine it. We couldn't either.

When I was a kid, I overheard my mom talking about someone who was allergic to tomatoes. No tomatoes? That meant no ketchup, no pasta sauce. I couldn't imagine. Could. Not. Imagine. Little did I know what the future would have in store for me 20 years later.

"In the Americans with Disabilities Act (ADA) and Section 504, a person with a disability is someone who has an impairment (either physical or mental) that substantially limits major life activities (such as eating and breathing and going to school), or who is regarded as having such impairments. In 2008, the

ADA was amended to include conditions that only show symptoms at certain times. Food allergies are usually considered disabilities under the ADA."[1]

I would venture to say that parents of children with any disability are just making their way, the best they can, at least initially. I would also venture to say that with increased awareness and education we can create more space for empathy and compassion regardless of the disability. I know for me, I just kept thinking, *if people understood this better it would be so much easier.*

My family's journey led me to learn far more about food allergies than I ever could have imagined. This journey also helped me find my voice, as an advocate for my children, as well as for the food allergy community at large. This book is as much a therapeutic release of all I've collected along the way as it is a space for connection and resource for others on a similar journey.

"I think we all have empathy. We may not have enough courage to display it." ~Maya Angelou

1. https://www.aaaai.org/Allergist-Resources/Ask-the-Expert/Answers/Old-Ask-the-Experts/504

Just One Bite

It all happened so fast. My daughter Shea was sick almost immediately from one bite of cake that we thought was safe. We always carry Benadryl and EpiPens, though we hope never to need them. Crying, vomiting, hives, fear in her voice and eyes. One dose of Benadryl, another dose. Over the course of 45 minutes, she vomited four doses. We had never seen a reaction present like this. Should we get her to the Emergency Room? I was trying desperately to appear calm, but inside I was absolutely panicked.

We were at my dad's wedding, excited to celebrate this special occasion. As always, we brought food from home for both kids and their EpiPens. We had snacks, dinner, and safe cupcakes on hand so our children could safely attend. When the cake was cut, they brought slices over to our family. I said, "Thank you, but no thank you, we have food allergies." The woman said, "Yes, I know. We were informed, and this cake was safely made for your children." What?! Really?! Wow. Um. Ok. I think. The kids were excited and they looked pleadingly at me as if to say "pleeeeeease, Mom!"

"Ok," I said. They took just one bite, but then I said, "Stop." This didn't feel right, I needed more info. I told them I needed to go ask about the cake and not to have any more until I came back. My husband, Jay, stayed with them while I went to find the bride. She confirmed that yes, the cake had been made specifically for my kids. "It is milk, peanut, and tree nut-free," she assured me. Yay! I went back to my family and said, "You're all good!"

But Jay said, "Not quite." He had just given Shea a dose of Benadryl. It was 2015 and this was our typical first step when one of our kids had a reaction.

Shea felt funny from that single bite of cake. "My throat is itchy," she said. These are the words she consistently uses to let us know she's having a reaction. Kids describe allergic reactions in different ways and parents learn the language of their own children.

It's easy to look back at the "shoulds" after something happens. We should have said no to this cake I had no first hand info for. We should have said no because there was no label or ingredients list to review. We should have modeled better for our children.

A day that was meant to be about family, fun, love, and time together quickly became a gut punch and life shifted into slow motion. Seconds slow as you assess your child's every movement, sound, and breath. We monitored her. I anticipated that in a few minutes the Benadryl would kick in and we could relax. But what we would discover over the next

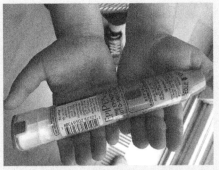

**Epinephrine
Auto-Injectors**

Epinephrine auto-injectors contain epinephrine, a prescription medication used as the first line treatment for anaphylaxis. Epinephrine is injected into the middle of the outer thigh. Each company has instructions on how to use their auto-injector. There are a number of epinephrine auto-injectors on the market today. EpiPen, EpiPen Jr, Auvi-Q, Symjepi, Adrenamclick, and generics. Regardless of the brand, people often refer to their auto-injectors as "epi." It's best to ask your medical provider for up-to-date options of epinephrine auto-injectors. Some require that you hold the auto-injector in place for as long as ten seconds, and some only as short as two seconds. There are usually videos available online showing how to use a particular auto injector.

Info/Videos on "how to use" epi products
https://www.auvi-q.com/about-auvi-q
https://www.epipen.com/about-epipen-and-generic/how-to-use-epipen
https://www.symjepi.com/how_to_use_symjepi

10, 30, and 60 minutes was that this reaction was different. More severe. Those four doses of Benadryl wouldn't help.

Ten minutes passed and nothing changed. She looked flushed. We separated ourselves from the rest of the party because it was hard to monitor her with others around who were starting to ask questions. We found a quiet spot inside. Our son, Thomas, was now complaining of a bellyache so we divided and conquered to help them. Shea continued to feel

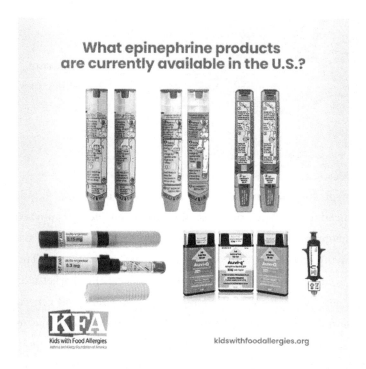

worse and there were still too many people around. Thomas seemed ok, so Jay and I asked my sister, Maura, to look after him so we could take Shea the short distance to my mom's house and watch her away from the noise and distractions of an otherwise perfectly normal wedding celebration.

As soon as we got to my mom's house, the vomiting started. We gave more Benadryl. Hives appeared. She vomited. More Benadryl. She looked blue. She said, "Something's wrong." Vomited again. More Benadryl. I had never seen her like this before and it was scaring me. Finally I said, "I think she needs the EpiPen."

Jay and my mom didn't agree. Her breathing was fine, so why epi? It didn't help that if you use an EpiPen you're supposed to call 911, which seemed like such a big deal. In hindsight, none of us were properly educated. Take the time to educate yourself – now. What a gift to those in your care, and to yourself, to be better prepared, just in case. I also wasn't convinced she needed epi because she was breathing ok and I wasn't really sure what else to look for when it came to using epinephrine. I figured that by watching for compromised breathing we'd know if she needed epi. It was scary and confusing for all of us, Shea included.

Finally, I said, "That's it, we have to take her to the hospital, NOW." My mom joined us as we set off.

What I have learned since then is that multiple body systems can be involved in anaphylaxis. "Anaphylaxis is a severe, potentially life-threatening allergic reaction."[2] Any

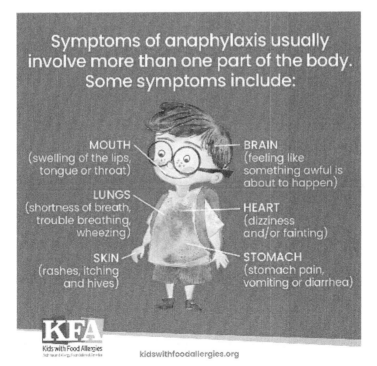

Symptoms of anaphylaxis usually involve more than one part of the body. Some symptoms include:

MOUTH (swelling of the lips, tongue or throat)

BRAIN (feeling like something awful is about to happen)

LUNGS (shortness of breath, trouble breathing, wheezing)

HEART (dizziness and/or fainting)

SKIN (rashes, itching and hives)

STOMACH (stomach pain, vomiting or diarrhea)

KFA Kids with Food Allergies

kidswithfoodallergies.org

2. https://www.mayoclinic.org/diseases-conditions/anaphylaxis/symptoms-causes/syc-20351468

severe symptom, or combination of mild symptoms, indicates anaphylaxis and epinephrine should be used.[3] Looking back, she had so many symptoms during that reaction. I would later learn (and be haunted by the fact) that not recognizing the severity of an anaphylactic reaction and treating promptly (i.e., within minutes) with epinephrine is a risk factor for fatalities.[4,5,6]

I sat next to her as we rushed to the hospital, one hand on her little hands and the other tightly gripping her EpiPen beside me. I didn't want to hurt her unnecessarily. I didn't know when it was "time" so I kept waiting. It turns out I'm not alone. A study done in 2013 showed that more than 50% of parents expressed fear regarding the use of the Epinephrine auto-injector.[7] We arrived at the Emergency Room (ER) and they took her right away. The doctor calmly looked at us and said, "Your daughter is experiencing anaphylaxis and needs epinephrine right now." I think I was mostly relieved. I think I had known in my heart she needed it but hadn't had the confidence to use it. So, yeah, I was relieved. I trusted she was in good hands now. Better than she'd been in ours.

3. AAP_Allergy_and_Anaphylaxis_Emergency_Plan.pdf
https://downloads.aap.org/HC/AAP_Allergy_and_Anaphylaxis_Emergency_Plan.pdf
4. Bock SA, Muñoz-Furlong A, Sampson HA. "Further fatalities caused by anaphylactic reactions to food, 2001–2006." J Allergy Clin Immunol. 2007; 119(4):1016-1018.
5. Bock SA, Muñoz-Furlong A, Sampson HA. "Fatalities due to anaphylactic reactions to foods." J Allergy Clin Immunol. 2001; 107(1):191-193.
6. Sampson HA, Mendelson L, Rosen J. "Fatal and near-fatal anaphylactic reactions to food in children and adolescents." N Engl J Med. 1992; 327(6):380-384.
7. "A majority of parents of children with peanut allergy fear using the epinephrine auto-injector." L. Chad, M. Ben-Shoshan, Y. Asai, S. Cherkaoui, R. Alizadehfar,Y. St-Pierre, L. Harada, M. Allen, A. Clarke https://pubmed.ncbi.nlm.nih.gov/24410784/

Within minutes her whole being changed. She got her color back, started to relax, and her blood pressure normalized. A drop in blood pressure is one of the invisible symptoms of anaphylaxis. Many people assume hives or compromised breathing are the only symptoms, but there are multiple body systems that can be impacted by anaphylaxis. Food Allergy Research and Education's (FARE) "Food Allergy & Anaphylaxis Emergency Care Plan"[8] is available for families (see page 224). This document includes lung, heart, throat, mouth, skin, and gut as systems that can show symptoms during anaphylaxis.

Before long, Shea was back to her usual chatty self. Thank God. Jay drove my mom home. He also went back to relieve my sister who had been taking care of Thomas since we left the wedding. I stayed with Shea while they continued to monitor her.

Once she was stabilized and settled, they set her up with a favorite TV show and the nurse handed her the remote control. She was so cute in this unique experience as a seven-year-old. She was excited to be in charge of the remote! "I get a remote all to myself, this is so fun! And I get this room all to myself and it has a sink and I get that sink. This is awesome!" She was back and enjoying every moment of the special treatment and undivided attention from family and staff.

For me it was a little harder. I was hit with a tsunami of emotions. Such deep gratitude that she was ok. Such

8. https://www.foodallergy.org/living-food-allergies/food-allergy-essentials/food-allergy-anaphylaxis-emergency-care-plan

heartbreak that she had to go through this. That *we* had to go through this. And if I'm being honest, I was extremely disappointed to have missed the wedding. It didn't seem like a big deal compared to Shea's safety and wellbeing, and yet it hurt. I love being with family. We had looked forward to this celebration for months. Much of my extended family traveled to attend; as more of my cousins were settling down and married with children, these gatherings were becoming few and far between. I sat in the hospital chair and pictured all of them together, laughing, happy, toasting, dancing, talking, and my heart broke a little. Not only did it hurt to miss out, I also felt guilty about feeling that way. I was on an emotional roller coaster as a mom. I wasn't sure what to make of it all and I felt very alone.

Then came the shock. How did this happen? I used to be an elementary school teacher, so I'd had training with EpiPens, and I'd been an allergy mom for almost seven years, and had managed multiple reactions before. What just happened? How could I have let my child down like this? My number one job in life is to keep my kids safe. I had failed to recognize the symptoms of anaphylaxis. I felt like I needed to learn so much to ensure this NEVER happened again. It was the scariest parenting experience I had ever had. I never wanted to see one of my children suffer this way again.

We got through it. We traveled back home the next day. The kids went to school on Monday. Everyone was acting like everything was normal. Once the kids were at school I broke down. I was walking around in a haze of disbelief. I needed answers. I called my dad's new wife and asked if I could please have the contact info for the baker. At this point we still weren't exactly sure what had caused the allergic reaction. I thought it would help to know. If we could learn from this we could do better in the future. But, after a conversation with the baker, I was no better off. She let me know she had not used dairy in the cake. I wondered, *Could there have been an element of human error? Could there have been cross-contact with the knife when the cake was cut?* I didn't push any further. I was no closer to having the answers I thought I needed.

A new level of fear set in. Our world had been rocked. Everything I thought I knew about managing food allergies suddenly went out the window. My comfort with the school suddenly felt threatened. In fact, anywhere my kids went without me suddenly felt threatening. If I couldn't keep them safe, how could I possibly expect anyone else to? How could others understand how easily this could happen? And let's consider the fact that both of my children have a milk allergy. Both of them ate the cake. Thomas had a stomach ache, but didn't develop the symptoms Shea did. How could two kids with the "same" allergy be affected so differently? Along with fear came total confusion.

Milk Allergy

A milk allergy isn't specifically an allergy to a glass of milk. It includes any product that includes milk or other dairy ingredients, such as cheese, butter, yogurt, cream, etc. The distinction can be confusing. In the US it is referred to as milk allergy, so for consistency I will refer to it as a milk allergy throughout the book.

I called the allergist's office and they were surprisingly nonchalant, "Ok, thanks. Describe what happened." "Ok, thanks. We'll make a note in her chart." The ER doctor had told us to follow up with our pediatrician because Shea had been put on a short course of steroids. We went in for the follow up and they were fairly nonchalant, too. I felt like I was in the twilight zone. Nothing about this felt normal yet everyone was acting so normal!

I did not know one single other mother whose child had experienced anaphylaxis. Jay and I had no one to talk to about it outside our family and friends. Nobody "got it." I have since learned there were support groups out there. There were people who actually got it, but I didn't know about them or how to find them. If this resonates with you, start taking steps to connect with people who get it. FARE has a search feature on their website *https://www.foodallergy.org/living-food-allergies/join-community/find-support-group* that can help you find active support groups by state.

Sending the kids to school was starting to put my stomach in knots. I started questioning how things worked and if they truly understood. I felt like we needed to reconvene and start over. Lunch. Snack. Parties. Halloween was just around the corner. I felt like we were starting from scratch.

As you will read, we learned so much after this allergic reaction. The wedding experience started to cripple my desire to "do the things." It took a while to get to a better place. But my suggestion to others is: do the things. Even the things that scare you. Even when it would be a lot easier to stay home and avoid. If there's a safe way to make positive memories with your kids, I encourage you to do the things. The memories are worth so much in the long run and if we're not careful fear can cause us to miss out.

Facts: Food Allergies and School

More than 15 percent of school-aged children with food allergies have had a reaction in school.[9,10] Also, food allergy reactions can happen in multiple locations throughout the school, and are not limited to the cafeteria. Care must be exercised during bake sales, classroom parties, and opportunities for snacking.[11,12]

9. Nowak-Wegrzyn A, Conover-Walker MK, Wood RA. "Food-allergic reactions in schools and preschools." Arch Pediatr Adolesc Med. 2001; 155(7):790-795.

10. Sicherer SH, Furlong TJ, DeSimone J, Sampson HA. "The US peanut and tree nut allergy registry: characteristics of reactions in schools and day care." J Pediatr. 2011; 138(4): 560-565.

11. Sampson HA, Mendelson L, Rosen J. "Fatal and near-fatal anaphylactic reactions to food in children and adolescents." N Engl J Med.1992; 327(6):380-384.

12. McIntyre CL, Sheetz AH, Carroll CR, Young MC. "Administration of epinephrine for life-threatening allergic reactions in school settings." Pediatrics 2005; 116(5):1134-1140.

Motherhood

My name is Meghan. I'd like to properly introduce myself and explain a little about why I've chosen to share my family's story. I was born in Boston, grew up in Connecticut, and am the oldest of three girls. When I was almost three years old, my mom was left blind in one eye due to an accident. My dad worked outside the home and we had no extended family in the area. My sister Maura was one and my sister Molly wasn't born yet. As a mom myself today, I cannot imagine what this must have been like. My mom tells stories of me feeding us Cheerios because it was so challenging for her early on in her recovery. Hard to know if it's learned or one comes into the world that way, but I acted as a caregiver. I still act as a caregiver. I want to help. I want to take care of those around me who are struggling, to lighten their load. I want to make things better.

This book shares the story of my journey into motherhood with the unanticipated management of multiple serious food allergies for my children. Like any parent or caregiver, I have always wanted what is best for my children. I want to help, to take care of them when they are struggling, to lighten their load and make things better. Many times, this has been out of my hands. I've had to learn to advocate, prepare, and trust. I've had to accept that through trials and tribulations can come hope and beauty. On these pages I share with you my family's messy and beautiful story of love and learning. If there is one thing I hope you will take away from it, is that you are not alone.

I was so excited to become a mom! I had dreamed of it since I was a young girl. My baby dolls had always been precious to me growing up, and my mom tells stories of me mimicking her every move as she cared for my baby sisters. It was an indescribable blessing when Jay and I brought home our healthy, beautiful, baby girl. Sweet Baby Shea. She took to nursing right from the start. Knowing this does not come easily to all babies, I felt extremely fortunate. All those late night feedings gave us time to bond. And all those daytime feedings too, which I couldn't share as she wouldn't take a bottle. At first it was blissful and all, but then, well, I really could have used a healthy break from my baby. By about three months old we realized she had to learn to take a bottle, or I'd never get out. I'd never been away from her for more than three hours at that point. She was in my arms for every feeding and it was beginning to wear on me. My husband, Jay, could also see that I needed a break.

My friend Liz was getting married in early December and I was looking forward to celebrating her marriage. I was also looking forward to an evening of adult company! It was going to require leaving Shea for longer than I had so far, so we needed a plan – and fast. It was suggested that we get her used to taking a bottle, ideally from someone who wasn't me. I didn't have a breast pump so bottling my own milk wasn't an option. The pediatrician had given us some formula samples though. Perfect.

We went to New York for Shea's first Thanksgiving. Much of my mom's family lives on Long Island and we were excited to celebrate with them and bring "the new baby." Since we lived in Massachusetts, it was always a treat to visit with extended family. We didn't get to see them often but they are a fun, boisterous, loving crew who always welcomed us with open arms.

Since my mom was going to babysit for Liz's wedding we suggested she practice giving Shea a bottle while we were together in New York. "I'd love to!" she said. So we mixed up that first bottle and I crossed my fingers that Shea would take it. I left the room because I had been told that "if the baby can see or smell their mom they will refuse other feeding options." Literally, my only concern was if she take the bottle. I had no other concerns as I left the room and my mom sat down to feed her.

It took her about five minutes to finish the bottle and when my mom lifted her up she noticed strange red welts on her face and a nearly golf ball sized lump on the back of her neck. She called me into the room using a relatively calm tone, but one that I knew to be unusual for her. My mom is a nurse. She brought the unusual rash and lump to my attention and we called Jay into the room. We were all uncomfortable with what we were seeing. What was happening? None of us had ever seen anything like this. She was only three months old and something was wrong. We decided to act fast and get her to a hospital. My Aunt Jeannie and Uncle Pat offered to lead in their car since we didn't know where the hospital was. Bless them. Jay drove me, my mom, and Shea to the hospital. They took her right in when we arrived at the ER. They monitored her and gave her Benadryl. After additional monitoring and seeing that the rash and lump had dissipated, we were sent home. I was relieved to get out of the hospital, but I was confused about what had happened. They didn't think it was from the formula, because so many babies take it. We had no answers. No recommendation to follow up with our pediatrician or anything. I was scared but I trusted the professionals. My mommy gut, however, told me no more formula samples.

After that, I borrowed a breast pump from a friend and over the next few weeks I started saving some of my own milk so my mom could use that to feed Shea when we went to the wedding. Fortunately the wedding was only about an hour from our house. It wouldn't require an overnight or extended time away. While Shea wasn't great with a bottle she did well enough that I was able to get away and enjoy a night out with friends for the first time in a long time. I was happy we found a way for me to step away and get a short break from the constant pull that motherhood had been.

Shea was such a sweet baby. She was happy and smiley, but she did suffer from red, raw cheeks at times that we couldn't figure out. The doctor suggested putting mittens on her hands and Vaseline on her cheeks. It was a mess but we did our best. She was a great nurser and super easy to travel with. I found that bringing her with me gave me some of the freedom I craved without the challenge of pumping enough milk to leave her. I always struggled to produce an excess of milk for her, so the bottle feedings were very much few and far between.

When she was about seven months old our pediatrician suggested trying cottage cheese "as a finger food" with Shea. Have you ever heard of this?! To this day, I have yet to find another mother who had this suggestion from their pediatrician. But, I trusted the professionals, so we did. Within minutes, all of the skin that came in contact with the cottage cheese turned red and bumpy with hives, as did the area around her mouth and chin. It was mostly "on her" but I knew she had also consumed some. She couldn't talk yet so certainly couldn't report to us how she felt. She seemed lethargic which scared me so I called 911. EMTs arrived and loaded her tiny little body in her infant carrier into the back of their ambulance. I was so scared. Jay followed us in his car. As if to add salt to the wound, the driver drove straight into a telephone pole across the street from our house as he was backing out of our driveway. My anxious mama gut could hardly handle it. Please! Get my baby to the hospital safely! They did and she was swept right back to the ER. They checked her out, gave her Benadryl, then monitored her some more. After a few hours they sent us home. That was it. Again, no recommendation to follow up with our pediatrician or anything else. Again I was scared, but I trusted that the professionals knew more than I did so I just rolled with it. I knew one thing for sure: no more cottage cheese.

Not long after the cottage cheese incident, I took Shea to visit my mom in Connecticut. Jay worked long hours and I often got lonely being home alone all day with the baby. Most of my friends worked or lived far away, and I didn't have any other "mom friends" yet. My mom still worked at the time, so before she headed out the next morning she did two of her favorite things... enjoyed her morning cup of coffee with cream and sugar, and played with her sweet "Shea Shea." Like any adoring grandmother, she planted big kisses on Shea's cheek. But unlike any adoring grandmother, within minutes her kisses left hives in the shape of her kiss on Shea's cheek. I had never seen anything like it. Neither had my mom, who again, was a nurse. We couldn't believe it. We quickly washed her cheek and after a short time the hives cleared, but we were confused about what was going on. Could the coffee have caused that?

It was scary. I wasn't sure what was wrong, but I knew something was off with my baby. The pediatrician didn't seem to be concerned so I decided to take Shea to a Naturopathic Doctor for another opinion and a different approach. The doctor used muscle testing to determine that Shea couldn't tolerate cow's milk. (I find emojis so useful. This is where I would use the brain exploding followed by the hand to face.) Like, duh! This made so much sense based on her history. She was about nine months old by this point and I was still nursing, so I began avoiding all dairy. The doctor also made the suggestion that we try giving Shea goat's milk as an alternative. It's hard to remember, but I don't think she muscle tested her for the goat's milk, which in hindsight may have made a difference.

I had no idea where one buys goat's milk. Eventually I found some at the store and served a little to Shea. Almost immediately she vomited, developed hives, and became lethargic. I called 911 and they got her to the ER. Jay met us there from work. They checked her vitals, which were ok, gave her some Benadryl, and monitored her until everything calmed down. But this time was different. Before they sent us home the ER doctor turned to Jay and me and said, "It seems your daughter has an allergy. Have you seen an allergist?"

Just stop. What? Time stood still. An allergist? I felt like I had been gut punched. HOW had we made it to nearly her first birthday without anyone in our medical circle suggesting we take her to an allergist? How had I not thought of this? I felt like a complete idiot. I was floored, grateful, confused, and angry – all at the same time. We said that we had not but we would certainly look into one, and thanked him and his staff for their care of Shea. Then we headed out, confused about what to do next.

Well maybe not that confused. One of the first things I did was call the pediatrician's office. I shared this "breakthrough" for lack of a better term followed by my disappointment with the care over that last year, and a request to pick up Shea's file as we would be changing to a new practice.

I found another local pediatrician very quickly. Next I had to find an allergist. Ahhh, I had so much frustration thinking about all the trust I had placed in the many different medical professionals over all this time. Why had I not stopped and thought for myself? Why had I not tried to learn more sooner? Some call it mommy gut, some call it intuition, whatever you call it, listen to it. Ask questions, try to get answers when something doesn't seem right with your child. You are their number one advocate, their voice. There are tons of medical specialists out there, but until you are in need of a particular specialty, you may not even know it exists. That was me. I had never heard of an allergist. This was uncharted territory for me, and I was totally out of my comfort zone.

I wasn't sure where to begin. On the recommendation of a friend who was also a doctor, I called an allergist and made an appointment. He was local, which was good, but he didn't specialize in pediatrics. At the time we didn't even know that was a thing – pediatric allergists.

Nobody prepared us for food allergy testing with a little one. Part of the process is what they call a "scratch test." They scratch or poke the skin, allowing a small amount of allergen into the skin as well as a histamine control. The more they are testing for, the more scratches/pokes. Then over a period of time (I think it's like 15 minutes but it feels like hours) they observe and measure how the skin reacts, while you remain in the office. An allergic response causes the skin to become itchy and/or to develop hives. They're uncomfortable and especially hard for a one-year-old who doesn't understand what's happening. They did the scratch test on Shea's back and told me to hold her arms so she wouldn't scratch. It was awful. I wasn't prepared for it emotionally. She was crying and looking up at me pleadingly with her sweet, sad, and scared eyes, saying, "No mama, no." I just wanted to burst into tears and give her the biggest hug, but I couldn't. I needed to focus and desperately try to find ways to distract her. I wanted to make this a little less miserable if I could. So we sang and I used silly voices. Anything to keep her attention off her itchy back. Since she was my primary focus, I 100% could not focus on what the doctor and nurses were telling us. If they gave me helpful information I sure as heck didn't absorb it.

After the scratch test they needed to do a blood test. Also, terribly unfun with a one-year-old. The combined testing showed she had a severe allergy to cow's milk. We learned that the protein in goat's milk is very similar to that of cow's milk, which explained her goat milk reaction. We were told to keep Benadryl on hand, given a prescription for EpiPens, and sent home with the small task of avoiding all dairy. Gulp.

As I've said before, trust yourself. If focusing on your child needs to be your top priority in a given moment then do it. Looking back, I believe I had a lack of confidence and underlying anxiety around being judged as a new mom that got in my way and prevented me from being a stronger advocate for myself and for Shea early on. Oh, if I could only go back and tell the me of yesterday that it's ok; that focusing on my child in the hard moment was the best thing to do; that calling the office another day and asking them to, "please repeat the information their staff tried to share with me but I was unable to absorb," is ok to do. It was a long time before I really learned this.

Pizza, Cake, Ice Cream

My fear became palpable. I was in near constant fear that something would trigger a reaction in my sweet baby. Threats were lurking in all sorts of hidden, and not so hidden, places. I knew social interaction was important to the development of a young child, but suddenly everything seemed dangerous. If we wanted to successfully leave the house we had some learning to do.

A few weeks after the official diagnosis Shea started a weekly playgroup. The structure included playtime followed by snack time. My little one-year-old was now toddling around, her independence blossoming. I was excited for this little human to be exploring the world around her, but I struggled with the obstacles I knew were there. Obstacles such as sippy cups with milk and goldfish crackers, both staples in typical toddler life. We were becoming accustomed to saying things like, "no thank you, not safe" as we worked to teach her and communicate about safe choices, but how do you help a one-year-old understand she can't have what other kids are having? I wasn't sure yet.

We started giving Shea all sorts of dairy-free foods, but I still nursed as long as I could because it helped delay the full commitment to food. She weaned at 14 months and we started to get in a food groove. Our mantra was: keep it basic. We made her food from scratch so there was no concern about ingredients. She was a great eater and willing to try just about anything we offered. Her favorite food was avocado. I remember asking the pediatrician if a child could eat too much avocado! She loved it so much that we used it as her "cake" for her first birthday party. We cut it in half, removed the pit, peeled off the outside, put it face down on a plate and stuck a candle in the top. She was all smiles. Strangest one-year-old cake I had ever seen, but she loved it! So much of parenting doesn't go the way we expected. I have found a hidden blessing in celebrating our new norms over grieving the loss of expected norms. No first birthday smash cake with frosting? No problem. Happy baby!

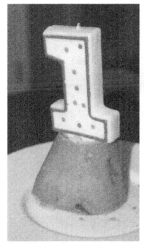 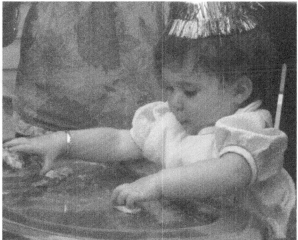

First Birthday "cake" and Shea enjoying her avocado during the celebration.

I knew she'd enjoy the avocado, but I also made a birthday cake. Over time I invested in my baking and cake decorating skills and started making safe cakes regularly for our kids' events. On a couple of occasions I was asked to make a safe cake for other people's children too. I loved it! But eventually it became too much and I put down my frosting knife. It helped me to know that where there's a will, there's a way. I was able to create some really beautiful, tasty, fun, safe options when I wanted to.

While her own birthday party was almost exclusively safe food, other parties weren't quite as food allergy friendly for us. Wherever we went, dairy was waiting. Care to guess the most common foods at kids' birthday parties? I have always said pizza, but as I began writing this I wondered if that was a fair assumption. So I did informal Facebook polls asking folks what they would say is the most popular food item and most popular dessert item at a kids' birthday party. Of the 68 folks who responded, 90% said pizza, 81% said cake/cupcakes, and 17% shared other food ideas. You get the point.

I get the point, too. These foods are tasty. And convenient. And not terribly expensive. I get it! If my child wasn't allergic I'm sure I'd be serving the same thing! But, my child is, so I have to look at food differently. "Breaking bread" with others typically means a friendly social interaction, and can be used as a way to bond. It's hard to socialize, bond, and feel included when you cannot share the food, when the bread everyone is breaking is unsafe for your child. I often had to consider the options and make decisions for my family regarding parties and food. Options like...

1. Say no thank you and avoid a party altogether? I liked this option because it was easiest. Definitely did it a few times early on in my motherhood journey. However, a time came when Shea was in preschool and the party was for a close friend. Suddenly that easy avoidance felt wrong. It was time to rethink how to approach parties like this.

2. Show up and see how it goes? Bring food and a cupcake that's safe so we could attend and she wouldn't be hungry, but it wasn't the same food which could be hard for my child.

3. Call the parents, explain our situation, see what foods they planned to serve, ask them to text me labels to review, or get the names of restaurants they'd be getting food from so I could call and speak with a manager to see if it would be safe, and then, if not safe, try to match safe food and bring that for my kiddo? Welp, I'm exhausted just thinking about it, but this was also an option.

If I knew the mom I would usually call, but I never asked them to accommodate my child. In our case, with a milk allergy, the food they were serving was never safe. Not once. (Remember? The most common party food is pizza.) Instead, I asked what they planned to serve so I could try to pack something safe and similar. This meant I kept safe frozen cupcakes in my freezer at all times. I never knew when a party would come up and I didn't always have time to bake. I also kept safe pizza makings on hand so I could make a pizza if there was a party. I hated parties. They meant work. Prepare food for my kiddo, spend money on a gift, and awkwardly ask

Silent Heroes

Sometimes people go above and beyond for you. It's a gift and I've started referring to these folks as silent heroes. My family has encountered a number of them along the way. Sometimes they are friends or family, and sometimes they're someone you hardly know. I remember a time when Shea was invited to a birthday party. I didn't know the mom very well, but she was aware of Shea's allergy. I didn't always contact party parents, and in this case my plan was to pack safe food for Shea and stick around if the parents didn't mind. Well, this mom took it upon herself to contact me ahead of time, and even beyond that, she insisted on providing a safe dessert for Shea. Oh my gosh, so sweet of her. I was out of my element though because aside from the safe cupcakes frozen in my freezer for parties, I didn't have a go-to brand. But she didn't even ask me for one, instead she asked about a brand she had found at Whole Foods. I thanked her for asking and said I'd look into it then get back to her. So, I called the bakery and spoke with the owner. She explained their process and it was clear that she and her staff took precautions around food allergy safety. I felt comfortable with everything she told me so I gave the green light to the mom. This was such a treat for Shea! In addition to the safe cupcakes they had a cake that wasn't safe, so Shea just took her cupcake first so there wouldn't be issues around potential cross-contact and accidental exposure to her allergen. What a gift to be safely included with her peers! The mom downplayed it when I thanked her. She didn't understand how different it was for Shea to not just be kept safe but to be safely included. I love silent heroes like this mom. She was a silent hero for Shea that day.

if I could stick around. Yuck. But, I actually got to know some other parents better thanks to this. And I reminded myself that everyone is dealing with challenges. I'd have my little temper tantrum at home, then get the food and gift ready, and off we'd go. The most important thing was helping my child safely participate in these opportunities.

I've talked to a lot of food allergy parents over the years and found there isn't a one size fits all approach to parties. It's often impacted by the specific allergy(ies), someone's comfort level with the hosts, their comfort level with trying new food, and so many other factors. Someone with a peanut allergy might be fine eating pizza and ice cream while someone with milk, egg, or wheat allergy probably would not be able to eat those foods. It's important to check ingredients and not make assumptions that food is safe.

Parties aside, it was challenging to eat outside our home. This was a journey on its own. It was nice when other people were willing to cook safe food for us but most people didn't want to risk it. My first "mom friend" was Dana Murphy. We met when Shea was three-months-old and quickly became good friends. She definitely helped with my sanity during those early momming days. She was along for the ride as we figured out that Shea had a milk allergy. Sometimes she would invite us over for dinner as a family. Her daughter Kambrie has a peanut allergy so I knew she understood food allergies. We used to do cooking nights together on occasion. We'd come up with a plan, buy the food, and cook together.

These nights were special for Shea because she got to eat the same food as her friends, which was rare.

Years later, another friend decided to take on the challenge of inviting the Neri family for dinner. Emily Grant texted one day and said, "We would like to have you guys over for dinner, so let's chat and figure out the best option. I was thinking tacos." Yay! I didn't have a "go-to" meal for other people to take on, because this wasn't the norm for us. So she and I talked and concluded that if we used Daiya shredded cheese instead of Mexican cheese, and skipped sour cream, it should be safe. And it was awesome! So many yummy parts to the meal including a delicious homemade guacamole. We enjoyed a fantastic taco night with their family, and everyone ate the same food! Again, a rare opportunity. The social experience was special and it meant so much that Emily and her husband Jordan took it on. More silent heroes normalizing safe inclusion.

My mom and my mother-in-law cooked safe food for our family from the start, with the added ingredient of love. Their efforts have always been appreciated. As someone who doesn't particularly enjoy cooking, getting a home cooked meal and a day/night/meal off was always an awesome treat! Jay and his family are Italian so there are a lot of classic Italian meals that weren't safe for our kids. I mean, manicotti, lasagna, baked ziti, ravioli, PIZZA. For family gatherings sometimes we brought food from home, sometimes my mother-in-law made separate safe options for Shea and Thomas, and sometimes they could eat the meal that everyone else was having. Always it required communication ahead of time, and a plan for the day of.

Restaurants were challenging. First of all, Shea used to break out in hives on her forearms and the backs of her legs specifically. There we would be, arriving at a restaurant, not letting our children sit until Jay and I divided and conquered with a package of baby wipes, cleaning every chair and the whole table. You can imagine some of the looks we got. It was totally embarrassing, but we couldn't care. Having our child sit safely was far more important to us. "Let 'em look and wonder," I used to think to myself. "Maybe they'll ask us about it and we can help them understand." We had far more issues at restaurants than we realized at the time. We hadn't yet learned about cross-contact (see pages 118-19 for more information on cross-contact). We didn't know that using shared cooking oil for foods like mozzarella sticks, chicken fingers (with milk in the batter), and french fries is what caused reactions when Shea ate french fries. We never understood why. Our go-to order for her when we went out to eat became grilled chicken, steamed broccoli, and a side of fries. Not too exciting when the people around you are eating delicious looking foods. Jay and I used to try and downplay what we were eating so it didn't sound good. Until we made the connection about the fries, as nice as it was to get out of cooking meals, a vomiting child in a restaurant or parking lot wasn't fun for anyone and certainly didn't make for a night off. The fun of it was gone. The ease of it was gone. It was years before we learned what was causing the reactions, and then we went out even less often.

A favorite gathering place for my dad's side of the family was a Chinese restaurant in Boston, called Royal East. After Shea's initial diagnosis I was really nervous about going out to eat. We happened to be meeting family there for dinner one night not long after. I asked to speak with the manager when we ordered. I had never done this before. I told him she had a milk allergy and asked what would be safe. He was so funny! He laughed, stood up straight, looked right at me and said "You've come to the right place! Real Chinese food doesn't use dairy. Maybe in crab rangoon at other places, but that's not real Chinese food!" He reassured me more than I can say. From that point on we favored Chinese food when we went out. The food was flavorful and the safe options were numerous.

When Thomas was later diagnosed with peanut and tree nut allergies I noticed that Chinese restaurants were being attacked in some of the food allergy groups I was part of. Why? Because they had peanut dishes on their menu, like pad thai, and other dishes with nut ingredients. I kind of scratched my head at this as I thought about it in relation to milk allergy. What restaurant would ever be completely dairy-free? Almost none. We had to be cautious anywhere we went. Butter was used in all sorts of dishes, let alone so many other possible dairy ingredients. For a type of restaurant to be vilified because they served nuts didn't sit well with me. Going

Resources for Eating Out

- AllergyEats | The Leading Guide to Allergy Friendly Restaurants Nationwide – Allergyeats.com
- Equal Eats | Translation Cards in 50 Languages – EqualEats.com
- Food Allergy Cards | Food Allergy Chef Cards – FoodAllergy.org

out to eat when you have food allergies brings with it some intrinsic risk. When it comes to restaurants it's so important to communicate with the server. I will often ask to speak with the manager. Straight up, if they don't seem like they "get it" we leave. We have done this before and it's only awkward until you're outside. We aren't perfect though. We have also ignored that feeling when it seemed like the server didn't "get it" and this miscalculation unfortunately resulted in a reaction one time. It was a scary reminder to trust ourselves. It can help to speak with others about how they approach food allergies and restaurants. Like so much of food allergy management, there isn't a one size fits all approach. We are still learning what works well, what doesn't work well, and adjusting with each stage as our kids grow.

When my kids were little, a couples night out with friends would have been absolutely lovely. However, we weren't comfortable leaving Shea with a babysitter so we usually stayed home. If we had a wedding or other special occasion we leaned on our parents or sisters as babysitters, but since we didn't live close to any of them, this was typically a pretty big ask. I was envious of friends who went out to dinner on Saturday nights. They would just line up a sitter and off they went.

That didn't feel possible. How and when should we let someone in? Eventually we did. I hired a young woman who worked in the childcare room at my gym.

I invited her over a few days ahead of time so I could tell her about Shea's allergy, show her the EpiPen, and let her practice with trainers. The gym didn't allow snacks for the kids so this wasn't something we had talked much about. I was a nervous wreck but tried to communicate calmly. Looking back now I wonder, did I overwhelm her? I would have loved a way for her, and future babysitters, to be prepared for food allergies without it falling on me. What if I forgot to tell her something important? How much information is too much information? The night came and I was a nervous wreck again, which made it hard to enjoy being out. I started hiring a sitter once a month or so for the practice of it. It got easier with time, especially when we found a sitter who was able to come more consistently. Less stress than starting over with a new sitter each time. Things get easier the more we practice them, so take that "thing" that feels hard and look for opportunities to practice. So much good came from this – date nights to keep Jay and me connected, a break from Shea, and a chance for her to socialize with someone outside the family and practice her routine with someone else. Experiences like these are what led me to create a Babysitter Food Allergy Training class.

I won't lie. There was a sense of loss as we found our way in the landscape of food allergy life. On occasion I would mourn, trying to process what it would mean for our future, our daughter's, and later our son's. Things would be different than I had imagined – our social life, parties and celebrations, interactions with classmates, teachers, coaches, and more.

But then I'd brush myself off, stop the mourning and remind myself to focus on what I had to do. I had to communicate about food allergies often, so I better get better at it. I had to practice how to set my family up for success in different situations. I had to keep my baby safe and happy, and wasn't that what really mattered? One look in her sweet little eyes and the stress dissipated. Being present with her made the worries and concerns lessen so I could remind myself what was important. I get to have this little person in my life! I get to teach her so many things! And, I get to learn from her! I looked for the small blessings in my life, showed myself compassion, then pushed on to do the best I could with the cards we had been dealt. Even though it wasn't what I had imagined we were figuring out our normal and finding our way. The more you practice looking for the blessings in your life, the more abundant they become.

Peanut Butter Jelly Time

A few months after Shea turned two we welcomed our sweet son Thomas into our lives. It's a special time in a family, having a new baby. I nursed him exclusively. Our pediatrician wasn't convinced he would have a milk allergy like Shea, but I was worried. At some point we tried a sample of milk formula we had been given and unfortunately he vomited, cried, and became red in the face. He wasn't allergy tested but we suspected he was also allergic so I avoided dairy while nursing him. We had also been given samples of dairy-free formula but he refused them whenever we tried. Apparently they're kind of gross, and since he was great with nursing I didn't have the heart to force it on him.

Fortunately I was able to get myself a breast pump this time around! This allowed Jay (or others) to bottle feed Thomas at times, giving me some of the freedom I lacked when Shea was a baby. Unfortunately, I didn't produce a lot of milk. I was constantly worried he wasn't getting enough. I had heard that pumping could increase production, but it didn't seem to make a difference for me. I did my best. I'm sure other nursing mamas with limited supply would agree – pumped breast milk is liquid gold, don't waste a drop!

Back then, in 2010, the recommendation was to avoid peanuts until the first birthday. This meant that along with avoiding dairy for him, we didn't give him peanut butter or peanut products of any kind. There was no such recommendation around nursing moms though, so I didn't avoid it myself. Peanut butter and jelly was an easy and quick meal for this busy mama. In fact, on many occasions I actually ate it for lunch over his head while nursing him. If only I knew then what I know now. Poor little guy. He had pretty bad eczema on his cheeks which didn't mean anything to us at the time. The doctor told us to put on one special cream, and later another, which was terribly messy. He scratched at it and got it all over. I worried about it getting in his eyes and mouth. It was tricky and the varied creams didn't seem to help. We were told to put mittens on his hands during naps and at night so he couldn't scratch, because sometimes he bled from all the scratching. I felt awful and utterly helpless. And yet, there's a high likelihood that my lunches were a direct trigger of his terrible eczema. Hindsight is 20/20.

I have since learned about the allergic march, or atopic march 19. Allergic conditions often begin early in life, and can first express themselves as eczema in young children. The progression from eczema to food allergies, allergic rhinitis, and asthma is called the allergic march.[13] It wasn't something our allergist told us about, so it went unrecognized by us as an early red flag. Both kids had terrible eczema on their

13. Allergic March | Allergy & Asthma Network (allergyasthmanetwork.org)

cheeks as babies but we had no idea what was causing it. I changed laundry detergent, cleaning supplies, soap, lotion, diapers, wipes, whatever I could think of *externally* that might be causing it. I don't remember thinking it could be caused by something internal, like what I was eating while nursing. I found it interesting that when I weaned Thomas, his skin cleared within a matter of weeks. It's hard to say for sure, but I imagine if a child presented with early eczema today, it would be handled differently and a lot of unnecessary discomfort could be avoided. I certainly hope so.

A week shy of Thomas's first birthday, Jay and I were going to attend my cousin's wedding. It was in New York. My mother-in-law, Nancy, and my father-in-law, Mike, agreed to come and watch the kids so we could go. They had helped us with the kids many times before, but this was the first time they would have both kids overnight. I left my usual long list of "instructions" and planned out meals for the weekend. An easy go-to lunch option for the kids at the time was sunflower seed butter and jelly sandwiches, since Thomas still wasn't old enough to have peanut butter. Out of habit I wrote "PB&J sandwiches" in my notes. When they couldn't find peanut butter in the fridge or kitchen cabinet, they found an unopened jar in our pantry, and made four yummy peanut butter and jelly sandwiches for lunch.

I will never forget being on Route 95 in Connecticut, in bumper to bumper traffic, almost to New York and worried we would be late to the wedding, when my phone rang. It was

Nancy. "Hi Meghan. Thomas has had peanuts before, right?" she asked. "Well, no he hasn't because they say to wait until they turn one, but he's going to be one next week so if you used some that's totally fine." I responded. "Well, no, it's not fine." She continued, "we thought he could have it because of your note but he is eating it now and he's not ok."

I felt like someone sucked the air from my chest. What? I started to panic, but what could I do? I was sitting in a car three hours from home, in bumper to bumper highway traffic. We couldn't get off the next exit even if we wanted to. I started to freak out inside but tried to stay calm while I spoke with her. "What's happening?" I asked her. "He's crying and the area around his mouth is red and swollen," she told me. "Ok, it sounds like he's having an allergic reaction. I'm so sorry, but I think you should call 911." We hung up and I sat for what felt like the longest minutes of my life. I desperately wanted updates by the second but I had to give them time to do what they needed to do. I called my friend, Dana. If you remember, she is also a food allergy mom. I cried to her, "I don't know what to do! I can't believe this is happening." She offered to go over and take Shea for them, which I was grateful for. Nancy called me back to say the ambulance had arrived and they were monitoring Thomas. He was ok at the moment, but they wanted to take him to the hospital for continued monitoring, so they were going.

I had never felt so emotionally torn. I was devastated not being there to help my baby or Jay's parents during this difficult experience. I was overwhelmingly grateful for Nancy and Mike and Dana, who all stepped up to take care of our children when we couldn't. And I felt so stupid for my error. Such a simple error in communication that led to all of this. Sure, I had no idea he might have a peanut allergy, but I never would have intentionally put them in a situation with a new food like that. I knew my children were in great, capable hands, but I was a mess in the car. While I was writing this book I asked Jay to reflect on his perspective of this incident. "I was worried," he said, "for you, for my parents, for Thomas. I felt helpless as well. I knew the best thing for you, for us, was to keep going with our plan. That turning back wasn't going to help anyone. I had to somehow communicate that to a freaked out mom. I also felt badly that Dana's family had to go into our home, given they had a child who was allergic to peanuts."

When Jay and I finally pulled into the parking lot we were mere steps ahead of the bride heading into the church, but we made it. There was no time to cry, no time to process. I had called my mom from the car so she was aware of what was going on at home and she'd told a few family members. It helped that some of them knew why we seemed "off." And off I was. I felt like I was in a total fog. My body was at the wedding but my brain was elsewhere. I was glued to my phone for updates. Shea was fine, having fun with friends. I knew this thanks to Dana's updates. Nancy kept us updated as well. Thomas was being monitored at the ER, had been given more

Benadryl, and would be sent home after a few hours as long as nothing changed. As a side note, I found it interesting that there was no mention of an allergist by ER staff. But since this wasn't our first rodeo, I knew better. I would be calling the allergist first thing Monday morning.

Once the wedding ceremony finished I didn't know what to do. I felt incredibly guilty not being at home. I felt like we needed to rush back as soon as possible. But Nancy assured us everything was ok. Everything was under control and everyone was ok. They didn't need us to come home and encouraged us to stay and try to enjoy ourselves. After discussion and deliberation, we decided to stay. But I continued to feel guilty. How was I supposed to relax, have fun, and dance the night away after my poor baby had gone through this?! And Nancy and Mike had just gone through something scary and difficult for them as grandparents! Often, the emotional impact of a reaction lasts longer than the reaction itself. I knew this from experience and felt badly that they were experiencing this without us there to help.

At some point in the evening I allowed myself a few minutes to process. Wait. What?? How?! We manage MILK ALLERGY in our house not PEANUT ALLERGY. I didn't know what this was going to mean and I wanted nothing to do with it. We were deeper in the club now. The club we never asked to join.

When we got home on Sunday I went right over to Nancy, embraced her, and we both cried. We bonded that weekend in a way few people bond. I was so grateful to her and Mike for their attention and love for our children and making sure things went as well as they could, considering. I felt like they "got it." They had walked a mile in our shoes, so to speak. The path for Jay and I as allergy parents had often felt scary and lonely, and I felt less alone that day.

It was official. We had two food allergic children, and a new allergy to figure out. I was scared, but, the reality was, nothing had "changed." It's not like we had been feeding him nuts and suddenly had to stop. Rather we were going to have to learn new rules to the game. Caring for these small sweet souls was our top priority and we didn't want to mess up.

An allergist appointment was needed. I don't remember how, but we were told about a pediatric allergist who wasn't far from us. We made the switch to him for both of our children. He was older. I took this to mean he was experienced. I made an appointment and the four of us went together. I was impressed by his staff. They took more time to talk to the parents than the previous office had. They even had us watch a video about food allergies. The only problem was, I couldn't focus on any of it.

As I have said before, allergy testing appointments for kids are hard. Shea had learned by this age what a trip to the allergist meant and she was not interested. Thomas didn't know better, but it didn't take long for him to start crying. It was scary for them and uncomfortable. It required bribery with candy, movies, and whatever else we could think of in hopes that they would cooperate. As a parent it's hard to see your children uncomfortable. You want to protect them and make things easier for them. We did our best to distract them and hopefully make the process as not-awful as possible, but after the scratch testing was complete they sent us to the lab for blood work. The day was exhausting. These appointments required mental preparation and some time to chill out afterwards.

Food allergy testing borders on barbaric, if you ask me. It's an annoying, somewhat invasive testing approach that can yield false positives, false negatives, and confusion about *what* they might be allergic to, *if* they're allergic, and *how* allergic they are.[14] They did a scratch test for Thomas that came back positive for milk and peanuts and they had decided to also test him for tree nuts. That also came back positive. Blood work confirmed he was allergic to milk, peanuts, and tree nuts.

While I could wrap my head around the milk and peanut allergies, I was upset about the tree nut allergy diagnosis. He had never had these foods. There was no indication he would have been allergic, prior to them testing and as far as I understood, there was no connection between peanut and tree nut allergies. Plenty of people can be allergic to one without being allergic to the other. From a daily life perspective, nuts can be a great source of protein and fat,

14. The article "Blood tests measure the presence of IgE antibodies to specific foods" covers 'False Positive' Results - www.foodallergy.org/resources/blood-tests

especially when you can't have dairy products. We "followed the rules" at the time and avoided them his first year but I had been looking forward to incorporating nuts into our diets once he was old enough. Wasn't it possible there could be false positives? Hadn't I heard something about needing to consume a food before the body can actually be allergic? But I wasn't an expert, I wasn't sure. All I knew is I felt bamboozled. It just didn't feel right to dismiss all these foods. I don't think they even asked us about testing him for them. So, I asked if we could try some anyway. I was told no. I jokingly said, "Oh come on, this is crazy. I think I'm going to drive to the hospital parking lot and let him try an almond to see." The response I got scared me. They said, "Mrs. Neri, that would be negligent of you and we would have to take that very seriously." Yikes. Ok this wasn't something I was allowed to take lightly. This wasn't something I got to have a say in. I got a pit in my stomach. If I wasn't careful someone could try to take my children from me. My only goal in life was to keep my children safe and healthy, and yet this threat lingered in the air. I had to accept the tree nut allergies.

We continued to go participate in a local playgroup when the kids were young. Snack time was even trickier with two young allergic kiddos. Your eyes can only be in so many places at the same time. I knew it was good for them socially, but I didn't look forward to it. I had to be "on" 100%, from the moment we walked in. My brain would start scanning a room before my feet even crossed the threshold. I would think to myself, *Is that a sippy cup in Joey's hand? What's in it?* and

Did Sally just hug Thomas and kiss his cheek? Should I ask her mom what she had for breakfast? and *Greta's fingers look messy and she's going on the slide with Shea. It's inappropriate for me to go over and wipe her hands, the slide, and the railing... isn't it?*

I can assure you that I would never *actually* go wash any child's hands, but it doesn't mean the thought didn't cross my mind. I didn't know all the parents, and it certainly doesn't sound very friendly to start approaching them with such questions. And while these types of questions made sense to me, I'm sure they'd have thought I was crazy. At least that's how I thought about it at the time. So, I just watched my kids as closely as I possibly could and cleaned their hands when necessary, particularly before snack time.

Utter mental fatigue. It was like battling in a war nobody else was even aware of. And the stakes were high. It wasn't lost on me that we'd called 911 multiple times in the kids' early years and that didn't count the numerous reactions we had managed on our own without needing to call for help.

Luckily we had friends in the playgroup from Shea's preschool. Those moms knew about my kids' allergies and became extra eyes for me. I'll never forget the day my friend Gina called my name from across the room, "Meghan!" while gesturing to Thomas who she had spotted across the room about to sip from another child's cup. Yikes! I ran over and swiftly grabbed it from his hands. I felt badly for any stress Gina felt, but I was incredibly grateful the way she made me feel less alone in a room full of potential threats. The program was nut-free, but had no restrictions around milk.

One of the things that helped, generally speaking, was that our kids' allergens were in what at the time was "the top 8." This meant their allergens were included in the Food Allergen Labeling and Consumer Protection Act (FALCPA) of 2004. It also meant we could trust that if their allergens were an ingredient in a food item, they would be clearly labeled on packaged foods. That said, mistakes happen with labeling and there are recalls for undeclared allergens rather often. People managing sesame, corn, mustard, avocado, for example, and other allergies outside the top eight didn't have it as easy.

I can only imagine how much harder it was for folks navigating food allergies before 2006. Even today, it is hard for those managing food allergies outside the top nine. Sesame was added as the top ninth food on January 1, 2023. It was meant to be a game changer for so many families, and took years to accomplish. I edited this chapter just about a month after the enactment of the FASTER Act because the reality has been terribly discouraging. Here is an excerpt from an *ABC News* article that came out January 12, 2023, just 12 days after sesame was officially recognized.

"Some consumer packaged goods (CPG) brands and fast food restaurants have already found ways around the new rule by adding more sesame to products and recipes so as to avoid potential punishment for cross-contamination with the teeny tiny seeds.

Food Allergen Labeling

"The Food Allergen Labeling and Consumer Protection Act (FALCPA) is a United States law that requires all food labels in the United States to list ingredients that may cause allergic reactions and was effective as of January 1, 2006. While many ingredients can trigger a food allergy, this legislation only specifies the eight major food allergens. This law was passed largely due to the efforts of organizations such as the Food Allergy & Anaphylaxis Network (FAAN). The purpose of this act was to prevent manufacturers from using misleading, uncommon, or confusing methods to label their ingredients. Someone shopping for a friend with a soy allergy might not know that lecithin is derived from soy. Now it must be labeled "lecithin (soy)" to help prevent consumers from consuming allergens."[15]

"More than 170 foods have been identified to cause food allergies in sensitive individuals. However, the eight major food allergens identified by FALCPA account for over 90 percent of all documented food allergies in the U.S. and represent the foods most likely to result in severe or life-threatening reactions."[16,17]

On April 14, 2021, Congress passed the FASTER Act. This amended FALCPA and starting January 1, 2023, sesame became the ninth major allergen that must be labeled in plain language on packaged foods in the U.S.[18] The nine major foods currently covered by FALCPA are milk, eggs, wheat, soy, fish, shellfish, tree nuts, peanuts, and sesame.

15. https://en.wikipedia.org/wiki/Food_Allergen_Labeling_and_Consumer_Protection_Act

16. NIAID-Sponsored Expert Panel. "Guidelines for the diagnosis and management of food allergy in the United States: Report of the NIAID-sponsored expert panel." J Allergy Clin Immunol. 2010; 126(6):S1-58.

17. Food Allergen Labeling And Consumer Protection Act of 2004 Questions and Answers | FDA - https://www.fda.gov/food/food-labeling-nutrition/food-allergies

18. "What Is Sesame Allergy?" https://www.foodallergy.org/living-food-allergies/food-allergy-essentials/common-allergens/sesame

Jason Linde, senior VP of government and community affairs for Food Allergy Research & Education (FARE), shared a statement on behalf of the more than 32 million Americans with life-threatening food allergies and nearly 1.6 million Americans allergic to sesame.

"We are disappointed and frustrated that previously trusted companies would rather add small amounts of sesame flour to their bakery products than comply with the intent of the FASTER Act, clean their lines, and safely feed members of our community," he said. "By taking this approach, they have turned their backs on some of their most loyal customers by ruining previously safe food, and made life even more difficult for our families."[19]

Managing food allergies has its challenges but in time you get into a routine. You start to learn the foods that are commonly off limits. You get better about asking questions. You find a new normal. It's tough when new challenges are thrown at you, whether that means discovering new allergies all together, like we did with Thomas, or having the food industry pull the rug out from under you as was the case for sesame allergic individuals this year. And yet, you learn, you practice, you adapt, you push for better legislation and you keep on keeping on, with safety always the top priority.

19. ABC News "FDA adds sesame to major food allergen list, updates labeling requirements" – https://abcnews.go.com/GMA/Food/fda-adds-sesame-major-food-allergen-list-updates/story?id=96370328

Pass the Magnifying Glass

It's ironic, really. Food is critical to survival and, yet, the wrong food has the potential to seriously harm our kids. Like any mom with two little ones, I was tired. I often felt overwhelmed. Regardless, I knew we had to keep dairy out of both kids' diets and nuts out of Thomas's diet for the foreseeable future. Keeping it simple was our first rule in food allergy management. We would most often serve them homemade food from scratch. Real food was our safest option. A protein, a veggie, a carb. Plenty of fruits and veggies. No macaroni and cheese on our table. No grilled cheese, no PB&J sandwiches. We discovered soy and coconut ice cream as treats as well as some unflavored potato chips.

I remember when Shea was first diagnosed with milk allergy and I was learning to read food labels for milk. It wasn't as simple as I'd expected. I had to learn words like "casein" and "whey" both of which are dairy proteins. As I mentioned previously, we were fortunate our kids' allergies were recognized by the FDA and fell under the "Top 8," meaning they had to be clearly displayed on ingredient labels.

Some companies make it easier than others. They might print allergens with bold in their ingredient list, making them easier to spot when looking quickly. Or, if milk for instance is listed in the ingredients they might also include it at the bottom with a "Contains Milk" statement. While extremely helpful, we learned the hard way that such precautionary statements are voluntary, unregulated, and should not be relied on.

I remember a time when I took the kids to visit my mom for an overnight. She was excited to make pancakes for them in the morning and had purchased a mix as well as some rice milk to use with it. She asked me to review the mix to make sure it was safe. "Sure, no problem, thanks for asking." And what did I do? I let my eyes skim right past the ingredients list to the bottom. I didn't see a "Contains" message so I made the (inaccurate) assumption that the pancake mix was safe and said "you're good!" One bite in and Shea said her throat felt funny. My stomach sank. I gave her some Benadryl then carefully read the ingredients list. Sure enough one of the first ingredients was buttermilk. I felt awful. I spent the next hour monitoring her to see if anything progressed. Fortunately her reaction didn't get worse that day and I learned an important lesson: read the entire ingredients list carefully! It's worth noting that allergic reactions can be different every time and with every person. There is no way to predict how a reaction will be.

Another time we were celebrating my niece's birthday. I was so appreciative that my sister Maura had thought ahead with all the food and ran the labels by me. This allowed Jay and me to relax during the party more than we usually could, that is until Shea came to me with her tell-tale line, "My throat is itchy." She had been snacking on salsa, guacamole, and tortilla chips. She said the feeling was from the guacamole. I was confused. I had checked the label. Then Thomas said he felt funny, too. That familiar pit in my stomach. We checked again. While there was no indication of dairy or nuts on the label, there was one ingredient that we weren't sure what to make of, "guacamole mix." We took them inside to monitor them in a calmer, quieter environment, gave them some Benadryl, and turned on the TV as a friendly distraction. Fortunately neither of their reactions progressed that day. Jay called the store where the guacamole had come from and after a few minutes of looking into it someone got on the line who said, "Oops, sorry. There is whey in the guacamole mix." Whey is a milk protein that our children cannot have. Were they for real?! After about an hour of downtime and monitoring, we rejoined the party, but they were a little slow and tired from the Benadryl. We were relieved it hadn't progressed to a more serious reaction but it had a negative impact on this day we'd all been excited about.

As I thought more about it, I was irate. How could they let this happen and be so casual about it? They assured Jay that they would fix the error, but he went back to the store a few days later, and nope. No changes had been made. None of the in-house-made guacamole labels included whey as an ingredient, and it still said "guacamole mix." He spoke with a manager about it, then stayed until they removed all the packages from the shelves. He said he felt responsible for others' safety until it was remedied. I was so proud of him for this. The next time we went back and checked, the label included whey.

When something like this happens, there is a sense of loss. In this case it was the category of "store-made food." As if the reactions weren't frustrating enough, now we felt hesitant about foods made on site, like guacamole. Fortunately Shea and Thomas hadn't consumed much of the guacamole that day and didn't require additional medical intervention. We try to learn from our experiences so we enacted a new family rule after this: when trying a new food, take one small bite and wait a few minutes to see how you feel. If you feel ok, you can have more. A reaction can be caused even by tiny amounts of an allergen, but we started to think about them going full tilt with a food they haven't had before. What if something is wrong with it? Wouldn't it be better to have less, just in case? Our goal was to catch any early symptoms and prevent a potential reaction from escalating. This worked for our family, but every family and individual is different. Not everyone would feel comfortable doing this.

Jay and I were still frustrated. I knew from seeing plenty of FDA recalls over the years that when a food has an allergen related mistake, there is a recall. We decided to contact Laurel Franceour, a Massachusetts lawyer who has focused much of her practice on food allergies. (I will share more about Laurel in the chapter "Tough Terrain, No Map.") We wanted to prevent this sort of thing from happening to someone else. She suggested we contact the FDA, so Jay called. Unfortunately, we learned that food prepared on-site isn't regulated the same way packaged food is. We were asked if our children had survived. Oh my gosh, yes! We were asked if they had been hospitalized with medical intervention. Oh my gosh, fortunately no. Since they hadn't been severely hurt by the food, there was nothing to be done. The store had done nothing more than make a mistake. Our optimism about enacting positive change and keeping others safer quickly dissipated. It became hard to trust the system and left us concerned for others who might not be aware of the difference in regulation.

While this was a disappointing experience, generally speaking labels have been our friend. This is good! Labels are meant to be your friend when you manage food allergies. One of our favorite allergists, Dr. Michael Pistiner, taught us "If it's not read-able it's not eat-able." Think of that cupcake in a baggie at the bake fair or that casserole at the family party, when you have no idea what's in it. Jay and I had learned how to read labels, and we practiced label reading with loved ones who wanted to prepare food for Shea and Thomas.

First and foremost, always read the ingredients label. Then, always read the entire label, don't just skim to the bottom (like I did). Precautionary statements can cause confusion. "May contain..." versus "Contains..." "Made in the same facility as..." versus "Made on shared equipment with..." What do these statements mean?! Well, if it says "contains" we get it. But what does "may contain" mean? "Such advisory labeling is voluntary for manufacturers. There are no laws governing or requiring these statements – neither when to include them nor what their wording should be. They may or may not indicate if a product unintentionally contains, or has come in contact with, a specific allergen. Likewise, the absence of an advisory label does not mean that a product is safe. Phrases such as "peanut-free" and "egg-free" are not regulated. Product labels can bear these phrases but be made in facilities where the allergens are present. Always contact the manufacturer if you are unsure,"[20] In my experience some companies are terrific about helping when you call for more information, but some are not.

It's also worth noting that labels can be changed at any time and manufacturers do not need to let consumers know. I found this very hard to believe at first! Sometimes packaging will look different which might prompt you to check the label, but often there is no obvious change. The best habit is to read the ingredients label every time, no matter what. Dr. Pistiner had also told us to use the "three strikes method" – check the ingredients in the store before putting the food in your cart, check at home before putting it away, and check once again before serving.

20. FARE - How to Read a Food Label - https://www.foodallergy.org/resources/how-read-food-label

In late 2019 I was contacted by a local news station regarding a story about Girl Scout Cookies and recent labeling changes. A precautionary label had been added to one type of cookie from one of two bakers licensed to bake for Girl Scout Cookies, and people were concerned. The bakery reported that nothing had changed. Nothing in the food preparation process had changed. The only thing that changed was a new precautionary statement added to the label. Precautionary labels are voluntary and can be confusing. Unless you call a manufacturer directly, it's hard to know how a food is produced.

I was asked to give my opinion on the subject. A reporter came to my home with her cameraman and we sat down for an interview.[21] I think she expected me to be all fired up and angry like others who thought this suddenly meant the cookies were unsafe, but I wasn't angry. I felt like this was a typical example of not really knowing about the product you were considering consuming. I believe this highlighted the bigger issue, a lack of transparency. I reminded her that nothing had changed about the cookies besides the information *provided* to the consumer. If someone considered them unsafe now, they probably would have considered them unsafe previously, too, *if* they'd had the manufacturing information sooner. Knowledge is power. The lack of a statement previously didn't mean they were safer, it just meant consumers were

21. https://www.cbsnews.com/boston/news/thin-mint-girl-scout-cookies-peanut-milk-allergy-warning/

less informed. There is an undeniable need for improved labeling laws. Families deserve transparency. They deserve to know what's in their food and how that food was made in order to make educated decisions. I recognize that families have different levels of risk tolerance around precautionary labels based on guidance from their allergists and from their experiences. I also recognize there isn't a universal understanding around some of these statements.

Precautionary Labels

Precautionary labels can be confusing. Unless the manufacturer clearly states that the allergen IS contained in the food, or IS NOT used in the facility at all, the messages can be unclear. For a consumer to have full transparency, their best bet is to contact the manufacturer directly to find out the process. And yet, there are no guarantees that the manufacturer will communicate processing changes with consumers, should their process change at some point.

My Crash Course in Precautionary Labeling:

Contains xyz --> This means the allergen is in the food.
May contain xyz --> We don't really know what this means.
Made in the same facility as xyz --> We don't really know what this means.
Made on shared equipment with xyz --> Ok, but was the equipment properly cleaned in between? So... we don't really know what this means.
Made in a facility free from xyz --> This means the allergen isn't in the building.

For instance, there were years when Shea only wanted to eat things that came from milk-free facilities. You start to learn which brands you can trust, and which you might want to avoid.

Food allergy management means preventing allergic reactions in the first place and the number one way to do this is by avoiding allergens when eating. Whether you manage food allergies yourself or you are a caregiver, empower yourself to be a great label reader. Practice at the store, practice at home, practice at the homes of friends or family. Just get used to reading labels and noticing how varied they can be. (There are a few examples included in pages 140-141.)

I can't stress enough that different families have different comfort levels when it comes to precautionary labeling. Some people will not buy or use a product that says it "may contain" their allergen. Others might call the company when it says "may contain," and still others might go ahead and eat the product since it doesn't have their allergen listed as an ingredient. It's important to determine your family's comfort level and respect the levels of others. My family's comfort level has changed over the years depending on our most recent understanding and experiences. Your allergist can also offer guidance as you determine what you are (or are not) comfortable with. Label reading can feel like learning a new language, but, I promise you, you'll get better the more you practice.

Doors Opening

Nearly five years into my family's food allergy journey my friend Keri shared an article with me. It was about an allergist at Boston Children's Hospital and a young milk allergic patient who could now consume milk products. What?!?! Had I read that correctly? I had never heard of anything like that; I didn't know it was possible and was desperate to know more. Keri hoped it might be helpful.

I contacted Children's Hospital and scheduled an appointment for both kids to see the allergist from the article. There would be a wait of several months but I trusted it would be worth the wait. Early on in our food allergy journey we had been told that many kids outgrow their food allergies by age five. Shea was already past that age and nothing had changed. While I held out hope for Thomas, I wasn't against exploring other options. Once the appointment was scheduled I often laid in bed at night imagining how different their lives, our lives, would be if we could say goodbye to their milk allergy. I could hardly contain my excitement counting down to the day of the visit. A group of my friends were excited too, as we'd all been talking about it since Keri shared the article.

It was finally time! Jay had taken the day off from work because we knew from past allergist appointments that it's much easier with both of us there. We piled into the car armed with lunches and plenty of safe snacks and drove an hour to the appointment.

I made sure to bring all of their previous allergist records so this doctor would be up to date on my kids' histories. I didn't want to cause any potential delay with the next steps. He took the records and spent the next few minutes quietly reviewing them. Eventually he said, "I see that your children have been patients of one of my colleagues. One of the best. May I ask why you're switching to me?"

He had to ask!? He must know and was just being humble. He must have families like us charging in daily.

He had the keys to our castle, did he not?! I reminded him of the article and said, "We want to do that. We want our children to be able to safely eat dairy and it sounds like you're the best doctor to come to."

What he said next absolutely crushed me. "I'm sorry, that was a medical trial, and it's over now. Your children cannot participate." That was it. No negotiation, no discussion, no opportunity. It was black and white and over.

We had gone to Boston Children's Hospital in the hopes that this allergist would change our kids' lives. When we learned it wouldn't happen I felt numb. What else could I do? So, we continued living the status quo and stayed the only other course; constant, vigilant avoidance.

My dad's wedding and our daughter's subsequent anaphylactic reaction happened about six months later. I'm so glad we were patients of Children's, because though I was utterly disappointed by the turn of events from that appointment, something unexpected and magical happened.

A few months after the reaction at my dad's wedding, we were invited by the Food Allergy Program at Children's to attend a workshop for patients and families managing food allergies. A group of food allergy parents came together in one room with renowned Pediatric Allergist Dr. Michael Pistiner and Pediatric Psychologist Dr. Jennifer Lebovidge, while our kids were all safely engaged doing activities with other staff from the food allergy program across the hall.

This was the FIRST TIME EVER that I was in a room with other allergy parents. It was amazing and I loved every second of it. This was the FIRST TIME EVER that an allergist helped me understand anaphylaxis, risk factors, and so many things I had never heard before WITHOUT my children present. I cannot overstate how impactful and positive this experience was. We were sent home with resources that I would later devour. I couldn't get enough. Drs. Pistiner and Lebovidge had collaborated with other professionals from an organization called Anaphylaxis Canada to create the "Living Confidently with Food Allergy" handbook – a guide for parents and families [AllergyHome.org], which they gave to each of us.

It was fantastic! It was the best resource I had come across to that point. In the weeks that followed I read it cover to cover multiple times to make sure I understood everything. I also contacted Dr. Lebovidge to ask for additional copies that I could share with other families or school personnel. The handbook anticipated questions I hadn't thought to ask. I felt reassured having something to refer to that provided practical information from professionals.

This experience was nothing like an allergist appointment. My kids were safely distracted in a separate space so I had the mental capacity to focus. It was a safe, supported space for me and Jay to learn more about our children's allergies. Dr. Lebovidge communicated to us that she was available if we had questions after the workshop was over. What a gift!

When it was time to go home there was a flurry of email exchanges among parents with the "it was so nice to meet you"s and the "we'll have to get together soon"s. I had high hopes of staying connected and there were a few emails right off the bat, but I could feel the magic slipping away. We all had busy lives and didn't live near each other. It wasn't like we could shoot down the street for coffee and conversation. My fear of potential food related accidents at school prevented me from traveling far during the school day so I didn't set up any visits. In a way I felt more alone than ever. Now I knew what I was missing: an in-person connection with other food allergy parents. Since moving to our new town we had only met one other food allergy family but it didn't seem that they were interested in connecting over food allergies.

I soaked up all I could from the new resources, memorizing as much as possible. I found it all very interesting. The more I learned, the more questions and concerns I started to have, particularly around school, so I asked to meet again with the school nurse and Shea's teacher. I asked some questions and they answered them. It seemed like they had things under control. I trusted there was a policy in place to keep my children safe and I trusted these professionals were following the policy, so I had no need to worry. But when it came to my children, I struggled to turn off the worry. I wasn't fully convinced they really did have it under control, which left me feeling unsettled. Oh, how I wished I could bring Drs. Pistiner and Lebovidge to the school to share their knowledge and wisdom.

SAFE

"Empathy is simply listening, holding space, withholding judgment, emotionally connecting, and communicating that incredibly healing message of you're not alone." ~Brené Brown

In the fall of 2016 I met Meghan Cassidy at a birthday party. Our daughters had been invited and as we each pulled out our child's safe cupcake, our eyes locked. It's a thing, being a mom who brings a cupcake. I learned that she was a celiac mom. I learned about some of her experiences navigating celiac disease. I couldn't believe some of their challenges, particularly with school. I could relate. Totally different diagnoses but very similar management challenges. We clicked in a way I hadn't been able to click with anyone else since our move to town. Our kids were in the same grade at the same school and we had both been in need of support. How had we not been connected by the school? Was it a HIPPA thing?

We figured if we were looking for support there must be others, and we wanted to find them. Within a month we decided to start a support group. It felt scary, but, at the same time, since what we wanted and needed wasn't available, this was an opportunity for us to try and make positive change. Anything we did would be helpful, so there wasn't much to be afraid of. I imagined what I would want if I showed up to a support group meeting, and channeled those feelings, expectations, and ideas into our early steps. If we could do it, you can do it! I knew from my experience at the workshop at Children's that connecting with other parents was priceless. We figured we could hold monthly meetings allowing people to share their stories, hear others', share ideas, recipes, stores, products, allergists, talk about challenges, share positive experiences, ask for advice, whatever was on their minds, and would help them feel less alone as a caregiver in general.

So we got to work. First was a name. We played around with words that had to do with food allergies, celiac, support, food, education, and more. We landed on SAFE: S for our town name, and Allergy Families Educating. It would be a support group for families in our town managing food allergies and/or celiac disease. Our first meeting consisted of four women in my living room, via word of mouth. A month later, ten of us met at a local church that had generously provided us a free meeting space. I couldn't help but think of the movie *Field of Dreams*. "If you build it, they will come." We built it and they came.

It had been nearly a year since the workshop at Children's. I was desperate for connection with other caregivers. I longed for a place to share my family's story with people who would "get it." A safe space to talk about our experiences and express all the emotions that come with them... sadness, frustration, guilt, confusion, or whatever emotion at the time. I wanted to offer that same support to others who had similar stories. Food allergy parenting can feel like a roller coaster of emotions. Each of us took a turn sharing our story. Part of me suddenly felt whole. Like finding a missing puzzle piece.

I had never met some of these women and yet I felt such a connection to them. I was tremendously grateful to them for participating, sharing, and listening. No two stories were the same. Some families have three kids, all with food allergies. Some have three kids but only one with food allergies. Some families deal with one allergy and some deal with multiple food allergies. Some families managed food allergies and celiac disease. We were all navigating different things. I found it interesting and was also amazed at the lack of consistency. There was no rhyme or reason to the likelihood of having food allergies or how they presented in a family. One woman was pregnant with her third. Her first two had food allergies so she was worried about baby number three. Would he or she also have food allergies? Yes, it turned out he did and they weren't even the same allergies as his older siblings. I felt for her. During my first pregnancy I never thought about food allergies. It was slightly on my mind for my second pregnancy, but after we learned Thomas had allergies, Jay and I decided our family was complete. I used to joke that "food allergies"

(continues p. 82)

Friends Who Care and Help

If you live in a family-friendly neighborhood, you know how kids like to bounce from house to house, yard to yard. Lexy and Carolyn helped me keep my kids safe in the neighborhood. They never fed my kids without first texting me pics of items and ingredient labels. They had their kids wash their hands if they had eaten something unsafe and were playing with my kids. They were kind to my children and I knew my kids would go to them for help if they ever had a problem. As I sit here thinking back, I hope I was as good a friend to them as they were to me.

One of my favorite Lexy stories was shortly after she had her third baby. She allowed Shea to hold him which was extremely exciting to an eight-year-old! One of the times she was holding him he spit up all over her. Lexy jumped up in a panic and said "Oh my god honey, I'm so sorry, quick let's wash this off, hurry, in the house. I don't want you to have a reaction!!" To which Shea paused and calmly asked "Lexy, did he drink formula?" "No, I nurse him." Shea said "Ok, it's fine then. I'm allergic to cow's milk, not human milk." We all laughed and Lexy was like, oh my gosh I never thought about that. That propelled us into an interesting conversation around some of the common confusion around milk allergy and how a lot of people think it includes eggs (which it doesn't) but forget about butter (which is included). This conversation gave Shea a chance to talk about her allergy in an informative way. I believe it was empowering. I was grateful to Lexy for caring enough to listen and learn, and for giving Shea a safe space to have conversations like this as she was growing up and becoming more independent.

Another fun story was when Carolyn and her family moved in. We went over to introduce ourselves and welcome them. We hit it off right away. They had a couple of pizzas on the table when we got there and invited us to grab a slice. We thanked them and said no thank you. This is the moment where I usually hesitate a little inside. Should I explain? Too much too soon? Or, since this is a first impression, is it an important time to be up front and honest? I chose to be up front, so I let her know that our kids are allergic to milk and cannot have pizza. What happened next took the four of us by surprise. From where she stood on the deck she yelled at the top of her lungs to her husband Mike who had gone back in the house, "MIKE!" "What?" "Can you hear me?" "Yes, what?" "Don't feed Meghan and Jay's kids, ok? I'll explain later." "Ok" he said. And then she was like, "Ok, we got it." We all kind of laughed because it was unexpected and slightly dramatic BUT she had just laid a foundation of trust for our family. She heard us and took immediate action to communicate the importance of that information. Friends who help lighten the load when motherhood feels hard are an absolute gift. These are just two funny moments but it was the years of support and care that I'll be forever grateful for.

was our third child. It required our time, attention, energy, and money.

SAFE gave me community. It gave me support and helped me feel less alone. I hoped others felt similarly. We were working to support each other and create a community we could all benefit from. I learned something new every time we met. It was helpful when parents of older children came, so we could learn from them.

In addition to a community of other food allergy caregivers, I had non-food allergy mom friends who were super supportive and kind and important to our family's journey. I was blessed with some of the best neighbors. Carolyn Rutkowski and Lexy Bulman did not manage food allergies with their own children, but they helped keep an eye on my kids for years. They were supportive of SAFE's launch. They seemed genuinely happy that I was connecting with other food allergy parents. They even came to the first SAFE meeting and I felt so supported by them. And yet, this was a place for them to be part of a community too. Through getting to know my family they had come to understand some of the challenges and could relate to some of the stories shared by others at that first meeting.

I loved watching things move along. We had a name, a routine of monthly meetings, and a space to meet. I really wanted a logo so I asked Carolyn, who is a graphic designer, if she would mind helping me create an awesome logo for us. I gave her some ideas and said I really wanted to include

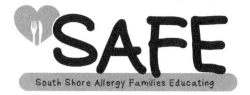

SAFE logo was updated in 2018 to
include more people in the community

teal in the design (because teal is the color for food allergy awareness) and she took creative liberties and ran with it. I love what she came up with, even all these years later. It wasn't long before we started a Facebook group for communicating about events, meetings, and anything else. Before SAFE, I had not been active on social media. Facebook made me uncomfortable. I remember Meghan C. and I arrived early for a meeting one evening and nobody else was there yet. She said, "Why don't you just do a quick post to say 'we're here, hope to see you if you can make it!'" Gah, the thought of this made my stomach flip flop. But I went ahead and did it because the reality was, maybe people would appreciate a little reminder and it would increase our connection for the night. I had to be willing to step up if this was going to work. Facebook was a way for me to step up. Like anything else, it got easier with time. I regularly posted meeting dates and other information worth sharing. Meghan C. was so helpful and encouraging during those early days as we got things off the ground.

I felt strongly about having a mission statement. As a former elementary school teacher I remember a professor who said, "Always know why you do what you do with a child." While SAFE was geared towards adult caregivers and not necessarily children, the significance was the same. Why were we doing this? If we didn't know, then there was no point.

So we gave it some thought. We were a support group trying to help families managing food allergies and celiac disease. We wanted to create a place for connection in our local community. Sharing stories was key because it's therapeutic and powerful. Maybe we could influence change in the community and help move the needle towards increased awareness and education. After spending some time on it we came up with "SAFE is a support group aimed at connecting caregivers and working to increase food allergy and celiac disease awareness and education in the community." Yeehaw! I didn't know what we would be able to accomplish yet, but I was excited for the journey. I had SAFE business cards made with our name, logo, mission statement, and email address. It was very exciting!

Aside from our Facebook group and a slowly growing email list, we needed ways to connect with the community and let them know we existed. The local pediatrician's office allowed us to hang signs in their lobby, a local Montessori school invited us to participate in an event they hosted, and we slowly connected with more families. About a year into SAFE's existence, a woman said, "I don't live here in town. Can

I still attend one of your meetings?" Oh my gosh, yes! The more the merrier, we told her! She said "Oh good, I didn't think I could." Yikes. We had inadvertently excluded caregivers who lived outside the walls of our small town. It became apparent that a name change was needed. So we became South Shore Allergy Families Educating, still SAFE. A much larger area that could include far more people. It was exciting!

We printed and hung flyers at local libraries, grocery stores, pharmacies, anywhere we could think of. It wasn't easy doing this on our own and I started to think that a website would be helpful as another place for people to find information, especially those who weren't on Facebook. Cost was a challenge for us but Meghan C. and I agreed to split all costs. With her by my side we forged ahead. We bought a domain name and website hosting account, and I learned how to create and maintain a website. This allowed us to have information about the group available at all times, and a place to share next meeting dates. It also gave us a place to share terrific resources including FARE, AAFA, AllergyEats, Beyond Celiac, and Allergy Home.

Our mission was to connect caregivers, but what about all those little humans who were the reason we were in this "club?" We wanted to do something for the kids. We planned a playground playdate at a local elementary school. A few families came and while the kids played the parents chatted. It felt like any other playground experience, but there were no snacks to be wary of. Playgrounds can be challenging when you manage food allergies. Little fingers with food residue on slides, bars, anything, can pose a threat to allergic kiddos. A food-free playground experience was unique.

We also organized a beach playdate for SAFE families. Moms chatted while kids played. We had to be careful about the water, but not food! Our gatherings were food-free and they were easy opportunities for families and kids to meet.

One year during Food Allergy Awareness Week we planned an event at the local library called "Little Kids ask the Big Kids." We invited two food allergic high schoolers to sit with a group of younger kiddos and answer their questions. It was a low key event with a great turn out. If nothing else, it was important for the younger kids to see happy, normal, big kids who had food allergies, too. One of the best moments was when a little kid said, "I'm scared of my EpiPen, are you?"

One of the High Schoolers replied, "I've had to use my EpiPen 16 times and you know what, I feel lucky. I am so happy I have epinephrine when I need it because it always makes me feel better. No, I'm not afraid of it at all." What a great message! When it comes

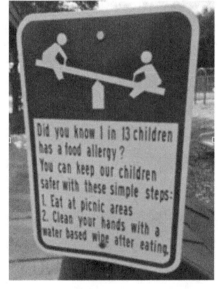

I noticed an increase in food allergy awareness over time thanks to playground signs that were popping up in different communities.

to epinephrine there is so much fear. Fear of the parents needing to inject their child, children fearful of this unknown needle they've heard about. As parents, we don't have the same perspective as our kids and to a degree we don't get it. For some of these kiddos it was the first time hearing from older kids who they could relate to.

We organized a SAFE team for the fall 2018 FARE walk in Boston. It was great! Kids and adults met up and spent time together. Some of us had never met in person so it was a great chance to connect and share our stories during the walk. It was also a totally low key way for the kids to be together. Again, this was a food-free event. It was fun to see teams who had been doing this for years, large groups with matching T-shirts and team names. Something to aspire towards.

After a few family friendly events we organized a "Parents' Night Out." A low key, adults only, get together outside our typical meeting approach. Some of the dads came! Up to that point we hadn't had any dads attending SAFE meetings or events. This was the first time I had been out with couples who all had food allergic kids at home. We could relate to the question, "Who's watching your kids tonight?" We understood what a loaded question that was and all the thought and planning that had to go into each of us safely leaving our kids to be there.

I often called restaurants ahead of going to see if they could accommodate our kids. One time while I was having this type of conversation I was connected with the manager and we got chatting. I told him about SAFE and he said he wanted to support us. He offered us a private room for our next meeting, and provided us with a beautiful charcuterie board. It was a fun, casual meeting of moms, many of whom had never been to a SAFE meeting before. It was exciting. Some of them had older kids and had been active in the food allergy space for years. Parents to learn from! They talked about the FARE conference (what was this I wondered?!) and 504 Plans (what do those have to do with food allergies?!). New connections were made.

The time came when Meghan C. stepped away from SAFE. I am forever grateful to her for holding my hand and jumping with me. Having her to launch the group made all the difference. She left a void. I knew the group and I would still benefit from having a co-leader. Immediately, Lauren White, a fellow food allergy mama who had been active in SAFE for a while, came to mind. She had experience planning events in her community and it didn't hurt that we had developed a lovely friendship in recent years. To my great satisfaction she agreed to join me in co-leading SAFE.

Lauren's daughter, Annabelle, had multiple food allergies and was close in age to both of my kids. As the kids got older, to our delight, they had a stronger interest in SAFE. We started thinking, what if we organized a kid-centered branch of SAFE? The kids could run it with adult oversight. We organized a meeting and called the group SAFE Kids.

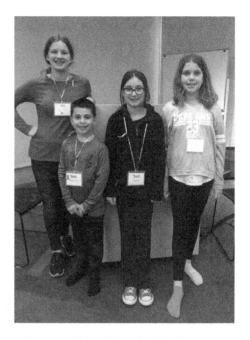

SAFE Kids: Proud moment for the kids at the end of their first event. Lizzie Power, Thomas Neri, Shea Neri, and Annabelle White

They were so excited and had so many ideas! Their first event was open play at a local library to bring families together and let kids meet each other in a low-key environment. They borrowed oversized games like Connect Four and Jenga from the library's Library of Things (so cool!) and we invited a local therapy dog for kids to visit with. We set up an arts and crafts station, and Lauren and I set up a table for parents and caregivers with information about food allergies. It was great!

That was at the end of January 2020 and, unfortunately, COVID disrupted plans.

As a support group, we had never had funding or a budget. If we needed something we paid for it out of our pockets. In the early years Meghan and I invested our own money. At times I wondered if we should become a non-profit. I remember a time when one of our fellow food allergy moms, Becky O'Toole, who was also a friend and local artist, sold one of her paintings and made a donation to SAFE. It was an incredibly generous gift and significantly helped with costs for our website and printing costs in the coming months, but could we just take money? Were we set up to do this on a larger scale? I wasn't sure, so we generally just avoided fundraising.

Lauren and I looked into starting a non-profit and in the end decided it wasn't the right choice for us at the time. A friend of mine who has a successful non-profit said to me, "If another organization is doing what you want to do then support their efforts, don't compete with them." FARE (Food Allergy Research and Education) came to mind and we wondered how we could better support them. We knew some families who had attended FARE conferences in the past. Lauren and I decided to go to the next one, in Washington D.C., and find out more about what was happening in the food allergy community at large and help guide our work with SAFE.

What a gift to spend time in workshops and lectures all about food allergies, current management approaches, research, etc. I felt like I died and went to food allergy heaven. These people got it!!! I could talk about food allergies all day long at the FARE conference and not bore anyone around me. Here it was ok. Here it was encouraged. Here it was magical! I met people from around the country, including Karie Mulkowsky, who at the time was FARE's Director of Education and in charge of FARE recognized support groups around the country.

We decided not to apply for non-profit status and instead applied to become a FARE recognized support group. This would make it easier for families to find us. At the time we met nearly all requirements, but we were going to need a

Medical Advisor. I reached out to Dr. Pistiner and he said yes. We sent our application off to FARE and hoped for the best.

In early 2019 we were approved! The benefits of being FARE recognized include having access to an annual stipend to help cover support group costs, such as our website and printing. It was such a gift not to be paying out of pocket anymore or hoping for donations from others. Another benefit was the ability to apply annually for FARE's Community Outreach Award (COA), which is basically a one-time grant from FARE. We would have to come up with a project idea and submit a proposal for funding. Such a great opportunity and I wanted to jump at it as soon as possible! I told Lauren

FARE = FAAN + FAI

In 2012, Food Allergy Research & Education (FARE) was formed as the result of a merger between the Food Allergy & Anaphylaxis Network (FAAN) and the Food Allergy Initiative (FAI).[22] According to their website, FARE enhances the lives of individuals with food allergies empowering them to lead safe, productive lives with the respect of others through education and advocacy initiatives and improved awareness around healthcare options and treatment. Their mission is to improve the quality of life and health of those with food allergies through transformative research, education, and advocacy. FARE has turned over $100 million in donor gifts into ground-breaking research and has provided a voice for the community, advocating on behalf of more than 85 million Americans living with life-threatening food allergies and intolerances.

22. History of FARE | Food Allergy Research & Education https://www.foodallergy.org/about-us/history-fare

about our opportunity to submit a COA proposal and she was on board, too. It was an exciting time.

We were able to provide educational opportunities for the community. Before COVID we did in-person events with speakers including Gail McNiece, a college consultant and allergy mom, and Amy Rose, the founder of a food allergy treatment program called Allergy Release Technique (ART).

Once COVID hit, we shifted to virtual presentations for guest speakers, including Dr. Margaret Vallen, an allergist outside of Boston, who also does Oral Immunotherapy (OIT), as well as our Medical Advisor, Dr. Michael Pistiner, who presented about managing food allergies.

Things slowed down for a while after that as we all figured out how to live in this new way, but eventually we resumed meetings, virtually. We used some of our funds to get a Zoom account. In 2021 and 2022 we were able to offer virtual contests, trivia events, and additional guest speakers. Our Facebook group remained active throughout this time. Learning how to pivot when the world changed was an important part of keeping SAFE going and maintaining our commitment to supporting caregivers and increasing education and awareness in the community. An interesting shift was being able to connect with people who lived beyond our south shore community. I heard from a number of people who had found our group through FARE but didn't have an active group near them, and asked if it would be ok if they joined us. Being virtual made it much easier to say yes!

It's funny to think back about FARE. It wasn't until 2015 when Shea had the anaphylactic reaction at my dad's wedding that I really started to research in an attempt to better understand allergies. That was the year I first learned about FARE, and I felt stupid. Had this resource been there all along but I hadn't thought to look for it? How had nobody introduced my family to this resource… allergists, pediatricians, other parents. I had not done much research online because I didn't even know organizations like it existed. At that time FARE was only three years old. Turns out, I've been watching FARE grow alongside my own growth. They've had to pivot at times based on what works and what doesn't work. The community based walks ended. The community based teal pumpkin projects ended. Support group leaders like me became the boots on the ground that families looked to. FARE became even more focused on fundraising and research. They continued to maintain a website that has a great deal of information and resources for families and schools. While I would have loved more in-person help from FARE, I knew funding for food allergy research was critical. Many of us were sick of this life that relied entirely on avoidance and carrying epinephrine auto-injectors. We had hope for a cure.

Tough Terrain, No Map

"Inclusion is intentional. It is about identifying and removing barriers so that everyone can participate to the best of their ability." ~Nicole Eredics

School was a place where we had to rely on others to keep our children safe and included. We learned a lot while our kids were in elementary school. Among other things, we learned to ask more questions, advocate for our kids, be persistent, and find the sweet balance between volunteering because we "had to" and because we "want to."

LUNCH

On Shea's first day of Kindergarten I got a call from the school nurse. "Hi, Mrs. Neri. I realize we didn't talk about this, but I went ahead and sat Shea at the allergy table today." Wow, that's great, I thought! This hadn't crossed my mind. Shea had never had lunch at school before, so this was all new to me. Since the school nurse had more experience with food allergies at school than I did, I appreciated her guidance and decision. I didn't ask any questions. I trusted it was all figured out based on best practice. For snack time, Shea's classroom was dairy/

milk-free. This made sense to us. At the time it was common for food allergic kiddos to be seated away from other kids who might be consuming their allergen. This usually meant sitting at a separate table from their peers. The allergy table. Some schools allowed allergic kids to bring a buddy to sit at the allergy table with them who didn't have the offending food in their lunch that day. This was better for socialization than the child sitting at a table with other allergic kids who they may not even know. But it's not always possible.

As an aside, someone once told me a story about a kindergartener who told his mom that food allergies were contagious. When she asked why, he told her that his classmate who has an allergy has to sit by himself at lunch so he doesn't give it to anyone else. Out of the mouths of babes. Children want to make sense of the world around them. If we don't educate them with accurate information they will fill in the gaps to explain things. Even if that means coming up with their own stories. We can do a better job of explaining food allergies and promoting safer inclusion of children with food allergies. At least, that's what I think.

The second or third day of school Shea came home and asked me what lasagna was. I started to explain but then I stopped and looked at her with a silly, inquisitive, head tilt. "Why are you asking, honey?"

"Because the girl next to me had it for lunch today and I've never heard of it." Huh? I did an internal head scratch. I was confused and thought I better touch base with the nurse if someone was eating lasagna at Shea's allergy table. So I called and told her how Shea said someone near her was eating lasagna. Then she said "Oh, well it's actually the peanut-free table so kids can eat food with dairy at that table." I'm sorry, come again? My milk allergic child was sitting at the peanut-free table, next to and among kids who were eating her allergen? This didn't make any sense to me, especially because she had been pulled away from her friends. The nurse explained that the peanut-free table was closer to her office, so it was easier for her to keep an eye on things. Ok. But that didn't actually make me feel better. She offered to create a table that was dairy-free for Shea. I couldn't fathom my little five-year-old having to sit by herself at lunch. Who knew how often other kids would have dairy-free lunches. I also didn't think it was necessary. Shea was extremely familiar with the fact that her food was often different from other kids. Preschool parties had helped with that. By age five she was already very clear that reactions made her feel sick. I trusted she would keep to her own food. I also trusted that she would be upset if anyone tried to touch her food and would let an adult know right away. Admittedly, I couldn't have 100% certainty about these things but we had to make a decision and, based on what I knew, I trusted that she could safely eat among her peers and that was the better choice than potentially secluding her. I asked the school nurse to please seat Shea with her friends and classmates from that point forward. She agreed and we had no issues after that with lunch. This had been the first time I questioned "an authority" at school. It forced me out of my comfort zone, and it was the beginning of learning how to advocate for my kids at school.

If it's confusing to understand why we supported an allergen-free classroom but not an allergy-free table at lunch I'll do my best to explain. It's about the amount of allergen exposure in a given space. Lunch tables and seats are washed after every lunch block, every day. In comparison, how often are classroom tables and chairs washed? I would venture to say occasionally, at best. If kids are eating snacks in the classroom without a hand washing protocol, they are potentially spreading food protein that remains on their hands within the small learning area of the classroom. As an example, maybe they ate nacho cheese chips for a snack at their desk (leaving a cheesy residue on their fingers), then went right to the reading table to work with the teacher in a small group. You can imagine that residue ended up on their desk chair, on the chair at the reading table, and on the reading table itself. By contrast, the trip from the cafeteria back to class allows any remaining food protein on hands to get wiped off, maybe on their lunch bag, shirt, or pants, etc., along the way. Kids eat their lunch then get up and leave. Snack time isn't the same because they usually stay in their learning environment.

We thought we had lunch time all figured out, and we were pleased with how well it had worked out, until a few years later. When we moved to our new town, the school nurse requested that we put in writing that we wanted Shea sitting with her peers during lunch as opposed to an allergy table, and to sign the document. I wasn't thrilled about this. The best way I can explain it is that I felt like we were being asked to admit guilt to something. As though, God forbid, something happened, they'd be able to say, "We told you so." I wanted to believe that if something happened they would proceed according to her allergy action plan: give her Epinephrine, call 911, and notify us.

Additionally, she required that our allergist agree to this plan of Shea sitting with her peers at lunch, and put it in writing. Since our move I had found a satellite office of Children's Hospital, allowing us to meet with a new allergist who was closer to us than going into Boston. We had only met him once so we didn't have much of a relationship yet, and we had never spoken with him, or any of our allergists, about lunch. In my experience allergists haven't bridged the gap between diagnosis and daily management. That part had always been left up to us. Even so, they wanted his input. I reached out and explained the situation. I was surprised that he also thought she should sit at the allergy table. I reiterated to him that her socialization was important to us, and we felt she could safely eat among her peers, primarily because she had already been doing it for years. I have to believe he was broadly thinking about the norms of the time. So I explained. I told him that she knew not to eat anyone else's food and she knew not to let anyone touch her food. He listened, then made the suggestion that she use her lunch bag as a place mat and keep all of her food on it during lunch. I agreed, the nurse agreed, and finally we had a plan for lunch. Agreements were written up and signed.

It was reinforced for me time and again that when it came to food allergy management situations, there wasn't a one size fits all answer. It was important to advocate for what we believed was best for our child, even if it went against the grain of what had been done previously. If you talk to different allergy parents you'll get different responses to the whole lunch table topic. For our family, we placed an emphasis on socialization while maintaining a safe space for Shea. Safe inclusion was our goal.

SNACK

As I mentioned, Shea's kindergarten class was dairy-free. It was common practice for classrooms to be free of the allergens of the students in a given class. Typically, letters were sent home to all families at the start of the year informing them of whatever the restriction was and requesting that they not send in snacks with that allergen for the school year. We fully supported keeping allergens out of the learning environment.

When Shea started her second year at her new school, she started getting hives during the school day. Frequently itchy and uncomfortable, she would go to the nurse and get Benadryl. One side effect of Benadryl, an antihistamine, is fatigue. She often got really tired, making learning difficult for the rest of the day. The nurse usually called to let me know what had gone on and we would see if she could make it through the day, but on multiple occasions I was called to pick her up so she could go home to sleep.

I felt tethered to the school. As though I had a cord that would only allow me a 10 minute radius during the school day. I had felt this way for years, but the frequent hives were only making this feeling worse. I hadn't felt comfortable getting a job outside our home since Shea started school. My "job" was to be available at all times in case something happened with one of my kids. Shopping at the outlets 45 minutes away? Nope. Lunch in Boston with friends? No way. Jay and I made financial decisions based on being a single income household. I realize it was a privilege to be able to stay home. A luxury to have the option. But it didn't feel like a luxury. I felt trapped. It was an invisible stressor. I've had conversations with other food allergy parents and learned that I wasn't alone. I know of families where one parent left their job because they didn't feel like they could trust anyone else with caring for their young food allergic child. I understood. People often didn't take Shea's milk allergy seriously. This was not to be malicious, rather they didn't "get it." They weren't aware and properly educated. Many times they could tell you about how dangerous nut allergies were, but had no idea milk allergies had to be taken just as seriously.

The hives concerned me but I didn't know what to do. Hives weren't new to us, but hives at school were. For years we had watched her get hives after her skin had come in contact

Elijah-Alavi Foundation

In 2019 I heard Thomas Silvera and his wife Ondina Hawthorne-Silvera speak about their story and their subsequent work. They tragically lost their son Elijah in 2017 after an allergic reaction at his daycare. He had a milk allergy and was served grilled cheese. The Silveras have worked hard since that tragic day to make a difference and to prevent such a tragedy from happening to any other child in a childcare center. They launched the Elijah Alavi Foundation, a non-profit organization dedicated to promoting nationwide access to diverse, socially equitable, and inclusive resources for food allergies and asthma in childcare, daycare, and schools regardless of socio-economic status or cultural background. They also introduced Elijah's Law which provides guidelines for the management of food allergies in childcare centers and daycare facilities.
www.elijahalavifoundation.org

with her allergen. Milk ingredients are in a lot of kid friendly foods so it had been hard for us to avoid over the years. Be it exposure to residue from ice cream, yogurt, or that cheesy residue from snacks like Doritos and Pirate's Booty, the hives were the same. They came on unexpectedly as a warning that her allergen was in her environment. It was disconcerting but we learned that by getting away from the exposure area, washing her skin, using an antihistamine, and giving it time, the hives would clear.

Hives at school were different because they were a distraction and disrupted her learning. We couldn't figure out why they were happening. The "Living Confidently with Food Allergy" handbook (you might remember this from the chapter

"Doors Opening"), put together by Dr. Michael Pistiner, Dr. Jennifer LeBovidge, and a team of other professionals, has a section on the three ways someone can come in contact with their allergen(s): ingestion, skin contact, and inhalation. It's worth reading to better understand. Reading this reaffirmed for us that Shea was experiencing skin contact with her allergen. For Shea, skin contact alone has never caused an anaphylactic reaction, but if the allergen enters her body via the eyes, nose, or mouth, there is potential for anaphylaxis. If my young child was coming in contact with her allergen then it was possible it could accidentally get into her body. Hives were like the sounding of an alarm. "Caution! Caution! Milk nearby! Leave the area!"

The contact reactions were having an effect on her learning as well as her level of comfort at school. It's stressful to worry about what kids around you are eating and what they are touching. Particularly when you're only eight years old. She was very in tune with having an allergy and knew to avoid her allergen. But we were confused. How was this happening? Where was she being exposed to her allergen? Was it on the playground? At lunch? During another part of her school day? Certainly it couldn't be from her classroom, right? She was in a dairy/milk-free classroom.

When fall conferences came I sat in the hallway outside Shea's classroom waiting until it was my turn to meet with the teacher. I saw a sign on the classroom door. "This is a peanut-free classroom." I thought to myself, "Oh, my gosh.

It doesn't say milk. That explains it! That's why the hives have been happening!" Surprised I hadn't realized this sooner and not exactly psyched that her allergen had been forgotten, I was relieved to have solved the mystery. It's much easier to remedy a problem when you know what it is. She was likely coming in contact with milk in her classroom. I trusted that once I brought it to the teacher's attention we could easily amend the situation. Finally.

When our conference started I let the teacher know. "For some reason the sign outside the classroom door doesn't include milk, which Shea is really allergic to. Can you please add it to the peanut-free designation and send something home to families?" She didn't discuss it with me, rather she suggested I speak with the nurse. So, I reached out to the nurse the next day.

To my complete and total surprise I was told "No. It's just a peanut-free classroom. Milk-free would be too hard for other families to manage." Whaaaaaaaaat?

I pushed back but she was firm.

Jaw drop.

I could not. Could not believe it, could not wrap my head around it, could not understand this. Neither could Jay when I filled him in. It didn't make any logical sense to us and we were not about to take no for an answer.

We realized quickly that we didn't have the support of the school nurse so we reached out to the Principal. After a brief conversation it was clear we didn't have her support

School Snacks

It can be hard for non-food allergic families who are trying to find school snacks that will be allowed in their child's classroom or lunchroom. It might mean they are looking at and purchasing products and brands they wouldn't usually choose. There are cases where non food allergic kids and parents have been spoken to by teachers or nurses because of food that came to school. I appreciate the schools checking for safety, but to what degree? Often, it's an innocent mistake. There's a fine line between promoting awareness and shaming. There are situations that can – I'll say it – make the food allergy community look a little crazy. I remember a mom on the playground venting about how the school nurse had called because she sent her son with a granola bar that was "made in a facility that processes nuts." When she said what class he was in my stomach sank. Her son was in Thomas's class and those restrictions were for Thomas. And yet, we didn't even have such a strict restriction at home. From the chapter "Pass the Magnifying Glass," precautionary labels are voluntary and not always helpful. Great, it's made in a facility. What does that actually mean?! Unless I call the company, I don't know, and unless Thomas was going to eat it, I don't have any concerns. The likelihood of Thomas reacting to a granola bar that *another* child eats that was *made* in a facility with nuts was basically zero. Yet this mom was called out. This was frustrating for her because she was trying. I called the school nurse to bring it up and to let her know that our family had no need for such strict guidelines. I asked that she please not enforce that on our account. It was too much for other families and unnecessary. We were grateful the classroom was dairy-free, peanut-free, and tree nut-free, which was sufficient and what we deemed necessary... a learning environment free from allergens. I honestly don't remember if the school lifted the precautionary label restriction or not, but I didn't hear about it again from other parents.

either. I couldn't believe it, but we pushed on. This was important. We reached out to the Nurse Leader for the school district. We thought for sure she would help us get this figured out. But that wasn't the case. After one meeting we knew we didn't have her support. We weren't sure what to do next, but accepting "no" was not an option for us.

I have often seen the suggestion for food allergy caregivers to "team up with the school nurse. They will be your best ally." Well, what do you do when the school nurse isn't your ally? How do you send your children to school each day when you don't have complete and total trust in the people charged with their care? This was a difficult time. Jay and I had no guidance or modeling of what to do, but we knew we had to push on.

We requested a meeting with the Principal and District Nurse Leader together (neither of whom still work in the schools). We hoped that ultimately this was all just some kind of misunderstanding. We again explained, "Our daughter has a milk allergy with a history of anaphylaxis. She is also contact reactive. She is in a classroom that has been designated peanut-free. We would like the classroom to also be milk-free to help keep her safe." "Yes, we are aware but this would be very challenging for the other families. We just can't do that to them." Ok, we thought. We would have to keep painting the picture for them of why this was wrong.

"The peanut-free designation for this classroom indicates that the school does not believe it can keep peanut allergic students in the class safe if peanuts or peanut products are brought into the room. Our daughter has been having hives from contact reactions since the start of the school year. We finally realized it's because her classroom is not milk-free. There are no hand washing protocols in place, considering this known allergen is being consumed. We are trying to understand how you think you can keep our milk allergic daughter safe in a classroom with her allergens if you don't believe you can keep peanut allergic students safe in a classroom with their allergens. What is done for one student should be done for all. If restrictions are too hard, we support food allergy education in the classroom and the removal of any food restrictions for the class. We believe educating all students on how to eat safely together is worth exploring and could be a more manageable option while still keeping all food allergic students safe. I am aware of at least one other school that has taken this approach successfully. Our goal is for our child to be safely included in the classroom the same way her peers are, and right now that is not happening. If peanut restriction is necessary then we believe milk restriction is also necessary."

This logic was so simple and reasonable to us that it was infuriating to sit and listen to them continue to disagree and continue to try and convince us why peanuts should be kept out but it was ok for milk to be in. We continued to push back. The meeting eventually ended with frustration all around and the District Nurse Leader agreeing to look into it and get back to us.

Over Christmas break and while we were waiting to hear if Shea's peanut-free classroom would become milk-free as well, I was able to spend time with extended family. At a family gathering I chatted with my cousin's wife, Danielle. She told me about their daughter's preschool classroom. There were no restrictions for snacks. Each child was given a napkin at snack time. They washed their hands, sat down, opened and ate their snacks, which remained on the napkin like a place mat, until they finished. Once finished they had been taught to pull up the corners of their napkin, so as not to leave crumbs, and bring it to the trash. Their next stop was the sink to wash their hands. She said it was easy, efficient, and worked. There had been no issues with food allergic students in the class. Another important piece of this was teaching them not to share food. I loved this! Safe inclusion without restrictions, through education. Let's be real. The FDA recognizes the top nine allergens but over 170 foods have caused allergic reactions.[23] If we ban all allergens nobody will be able to eat anything. I think it's important to explore options like this for long term safety and sustainability. You eat your snack, I eat my snack, nobody shares. It might feel like this goes against teaching young children the important skill of sharing, but we can teach them the difference when it comes to food at school. Kids are smart and will learn if we help teach them. She helped me believe there was hope with proper education.

23. NIAID-Sponsored Expert Panel. "Guidelines for the diagnosis and management of food allergy in the United States: Report of the NIAID-sponsored expert panel." J Allergy Clin Immunol. 2010; 126(6):51- 58.

PARTIES

Before becoming a food allergy parent, I didn't think much about food at school, but once I became a food allergy parent, every type of food use mattered. Who was making decisions and how were they made? What did I have to worry about and when could I let my guard down? As I learned from working with multiple schools over the years, there wasn't a one size fits all approach.

My experience with classroom parties went back as far as my own childhood with school celebrations (which included dunking for apples after eating a donut off a string), then to class parties when I was a teacher, then when I would attend as a mom, and eventually when I participated as a room parent. I've seen parents prepare some pretty amazing "party food" – cake pops, cupcakes, cakes, cookies. You only need to do a quick Pinterest search to see all the creative ways food can be prepared.

Our new school district adopted a wellness policy a year or two prior to our arrival that, among other things, restricted unhealthy food from classroom celebrations. This meant no more of the traditional "party food," a step away from all those Pinterest worthy cakes and cupcakes. I appreciated a step towards wellness but had to bear in mind that healthy did not equal safe. I had some concern about the safety of some of the foods, particularly those prepared in people's homes. With junk food options off the table I noticed a creative coordination of healthy food items at our new school; fun shaped fruit salad, popcorn in cute containers, and more. Parents were working hard to keep the food fun and memorable which was great! Unfortunately, when party time came, kids often took a bite or two then dumped the rest in the trash.

So, is it for the kids? How much do they really care? Is food what brings the fun? After a few challenging parties in our new school and having experienced a successful approach at our previous school, I had come to two conclusions. First, the coordination of shared food is not necessary and second, we can move the focus from food to fun. I figured, why not shoot for the moon and try for both!

Our previous school had introduced something called "Party in a Bag." I don't know who started it or why, but it was fantastic for food allergy families because it eliminated shared food! Each child in the class was given a paper lunch bag a few days ahead of the classroom celebration. A limited amount of classroom time was used to decorate the bag, then it was sent home with a note inside asking caregivers to fill it with "something salty, something sweet, and something to drink." This would be their food during the classroom celebration. There were some early concerns about kids forgetting it at home, or some kids having amazingly fancy items while others had "eh" items, but it worked out well in the end. Room parents always put together extra bags in case anyone forgot theirs, including allergy friendly bags based on known allergens. It was a basic snack. Most parents and caregivers didn't go beyond what they typically packed for snack. That way it wasn't an added stressor for them. But, it was more fun for the kids when it came out of their "special" bag.

I missed this approach, which contributed to my uneasiness with parties following Shea's reaction at my dad's wedding. The idea of shared food really stressed me out, and Halloween was around the corner. I was talking to a neighbor one morning after getting the kids to school. She asked how the kids were adjusting to town and their new school. Their food allergies came up and I shared my stress about the upcoming classroom celebrations, along with the Party in a Bag idea from our previous school. She was encouraging, saying that I might be able to influence change in this school district if I shared the idea. She gave me the name of the school district's Chair of Health and Wellness, so I reached out to him.

Each month the Health and Wellness Chair led a Healthy Elementary Schools Task Force meeting for families and staff of the school district, and it just so happened his next meeting was that very afternoon. He invited me to attend and share my idea. Yay! I really appreciated the opportunity to share it and promote awareness, but I was unclear on next steps for actually implementing this alternative approach to party food.

The meeting consisted primarily of fellow parents, none of whom identified themselves as food allergy parents. At the end of the meeting a woman stopped me and said she thought the idea was great and she'd be happy to go with me to speak with principals and nurses at each of our town's four elementary schools. It was just the push I needed and gave me a next step. Over the coming days and weeks we made appointments and did a district tour. We were met with smiles and "thank you"s and "that's a nice idea" but nobody seemed interested in *actually* moving forward with the idea.

I discovered it wasn't that simple. Food use at parties was up to individual room parents, determined by the PTO (Parent Teacher Organization), at individual schools for individual classrooms. There are four elementary schools in our town with multiple classrooms at each grade level. Things suddenly felt overwhelming. I remember bumping into the PTO President from one of the other schools at the grocery store one day. I ran the Party in a Bag idea by her but she didn't seem interested. Silly me. I had expected people to gravitate to this idea, but they didn't. I hadn't found anyone who was interested in moving forward with it and I couldn't fathom tracking down each room parent at each school. What I could fathom was trying to advocate for the food allergic community at my own children's school, so I started attending PTO meetings. I didn't want to seem pushy. I floated the idea out there but no bites. The Halloween party came and went with shared food for the kids. Then a winter Holiday party, a Valentine's Day party, followed by a variety of spring celebrations. It was fine. That is, if fine means having anxiety for the week leading up to an event and clearing your calendar to ensure you can attend. Yeah, totally fine.

Since room parents coordinated snacks and activities for classroom parties, I joined the PTO and signed up to be a Room Parent. Since I wanted to see if we could stop the coordination of shared food I brought up the "Party in a Bag" idea at a PTO meeting. It wasn't disparaged but it also wasn't celebrated. No matter how hard I tried, there just wasn't much interest in it. Ok, I thought. What if I model it just in my child's class? If it goes well then maybe it will catch on. As a co-room parent that year I couldn't wait to share this idea with the other mom. I was excited for us to give it a try.

But the joke was on me. She wasn't interested at all! After I explained the idea she coolly replied, "No. I'd rather not do that." The wind was sucked from my sails. Seriously? It felt like I was trying to sprint through mud and couldn't get traction. To make the changes I was hoping to make I was at the mercy of other people's willingness, which was incredibly frustrating and discouraging when they weren't willing to give things a go.

She had no issues keeping all food safe, but she couldn't step away from the coordination of shared food. When you don't live this life it's hard to understand the anxiety that can come with it. It's hard to explain to someone who doesn't understand food allergy anxiety that giving your child a new food for the first time during a school party isn't ideal. It probably sounded crazy to her and honestly, I hated having these kinds of awkward conversations anyway. It left room for judgment.

One of the best surprises was finding out that a few friends, who were room parents in other classrooms, ran with the Party In a Bag idea. At least I could live vicariously through them! They were piloting the approach for me. The feedback was great. It sounded like coordinating parties was easier. They provided the bags, made sure to have a few extras on hand in case kids forgot, and then just found a fun activity to do with the class. Without support from higher up, however, it didn't last. I took a step back the following year, feeling deflated and discouraged. While my preference was that we stop making decisions about what other people's kids eat, I had to accept that change is hard. For the time being, shared food was still a party priority.

Sharing Food

Other reasons that shared food isn't ideal: some kids have sensitivities that aren't treated the same way allergies are so there would be no attempt to eliminate foods they really can't eat. Some children, for religious or other reasons, don't eat certain things. Avoiding shared food means they aren't singled out or left out. Food restrictions are hard in social settings, regardless of why there is a restriction. I don't think school should be a place where kids have to worry about the food they can or cannot eat, even if it's not life-threatening. Private gatherings are completely different, where hosts will make their own decisions.

Moving from food to fun was also something that wasn't about to happen quickly. Food was the primary focus of most of the parties I had attended. What if we focus on the idea of fun for a minute? How many kids do you know who like to have fun?! I know lots of them! How many kids do you know who might benefit from the focus being taken off food? Plenty of kids! If you were to coordinate a party with fun activities, is it possible those activities could outweigh the food? In my opinion, yes!

I remember a Valentine's Day party when I reached out to the room moms ahead of time (I was not a room parent at the time). I thought touching base in advance would be the best way to get a heads up about food that was planned for the party so I would know to be prepared with something else if necessary. I also thought it might allow me the chance to share some fun activity ideas. They said they didn't need any help with planning but I was welcome to attend. Darn. I didn't get very far. I had been noticing parties becoming more and more about the food so I decided to initiate a little "Operation Party Fun" on my own. Ahead of the party I prepared a simple, fun activity. I knew from experience as an elementary school teacher that it is good to have backup plans. There was a good chance we wouldn't do it, but I felt compelled to bring something. My activity entailed a bunch of little red paper hearts and some tape. That was it. While the kids had their snack I discreetly hid 20 hearts around the classroom. When they finished their Wellness Policy approved party food (one or two bites, trash) there was nothing to do. As I had anticipated, "snack time" was the party activity. So I quietly jumped into action. As they finished, I whispered individually, "There are 20 little red hearts hidden around the room. Quietly, so you don't give it away to your classmates, why don't you wander the room and see how many you can find." It was great. They were happy to have something to do, and were quiet and well behaved so it wasn't disruptive. In my experience any kind of scavenger hunt is fun for elementary aged children.

Before leaving I took down all the hearts, no mess left behind. It wasn't complicated. I do think there can be a lot of pressure on room parents to come up with "amazing parties" for the kids, both food and activities. That can be intimidating. There are ways to keep it simple and fun. Kids love to have fun so why not enlist them at the start of the year by asking for ideas that don't require much in the way of prep or materials (freeze dance, musical chairs, scavenger hunts, seven-up and plenty of other games)? You can also set up make-and-take stations with plain paper and some markers for them to make someone a card for instance. Maybe they'll challenge themselves to come up with a cute poem for the card. Simple. A break from their typical school routine. Let's take some pressure off the parents planning these events, and keep food for nourishment rather than entertainment. You can find more food-free fun ideas on pages 242-243.

FIELD DAY

In addition to lunch, snacks, and parties, there were also the once a year annual or random school-wide events that I had to navigate. Field Day was one such event. With the Wellness Policy in place, field day moved from popsicles and other snacks, to cut up fruit. Back when Jay and I attended the workshop at Children's Hospital we learned that cutting boards can be sources of cross-contact (see pages 118-119 for helpful resources from FoodAllergy.org). Consider this: if someone cuts cheese on a cutting board then cuts fruit without washing in between, small amounts of the cheese can remain, which could cause an allergic reaction if a milk allergic individual eats the fruit. While cross-contact is unintended, it only takes a small amount of an allergen to cause a reaction.

When it came to food use at school I was discovering a gray area around "safe" food. My comfort zone wasn't in line with the rules of the school. Fruit salad met the Wellness Policy as healthy, and in theory was "safe," but how were we to know about the potential for cross-contact? We had no way of knowing. When I would reach out to the nurse, principal, or district nurse leader for support I was told more than once "you have no idea how far we've come." They were alluding to the Wellness Policy and the changes that had already been made district wide regarding events and celebrations. While I appreciated the progress, ultimately I didn't find this particularly helpful, forward thinking, or acceptable. Was I not allowed to want better? To improve further? As far as I was concerned there was still work to be done and I really wanted the support of these important individuals. In the meantime it was business as usual and I couldn't let my guard down.

This wouldn't be the fault of volunteering parents so I mean no disrespect here. It was never brought up and volunteers who provided food for school events were given no guidance or training on safe preparation with regard to food allergies. In my experience people usually want to be helpful, but they need information and guidance. Without that, something as benign as fruit salad can pose a threat.

This was the issue with Field Day. Field Day is a school wide event with over 20 stations of fun physical activities outside. Classes visit each station over the course of the day. It's usually at the end of the school year, which in New England often means it's warm and sunny. The kids get a lunch break between their morning and afternoon Field Day sessions. They are provided with refreshments at snack tents. Parents donated healthy and "safe" cut up oranges and watermelon for the kids during these breaks. Healthy yes, but unfortunately posing a possible risk of cross-contact. It was a risk I wasn't willing to take with my kids. As I said, there had been no training around food allergy safe food prep so people who didn't live with allergies couldn't be expected to understand how to avoid cross-contact. As a food allergy parent it can be an uncomfortable topic. You worry it's like you're accusing others of not being clean enough. This isn't it. We know how easy it is for things to happen that can put our kids at risk. Food allergies are zero tolerance. As parents we are well aware you don't get credit for "trying" after a reaction happens. We look at everything with a different eye. So, I cut fruit at home, packaged it clearly, kept it cold, then ran around like a crazy woman during Field Day to find both kids and make sure they had their safe snack when their class took a refreshment break.

Prevent Cross-Contact

Keep diners with food allergies safe. Even a tiny amount of an allergen can cause a severe and potentially life-threatening allergic reaction.

Cross-Contact	Cross-Contamination
Occurs when an allergen is unintentionally transferred from one food to another	Occurs when microorganisms like bacteria contaminate food
Can cause food allergy reactions	Can cause foodborne illnesses
Proper cooking does NOT reduce or eliminate the chances of a food allergy reaction	Proper cooking may reduce or eliminate the chances of foodborne illness

 Always wash hands and change gloves between preparing different menu items

 Clean and sanitize surfaces between every menu item: countertops, cutting boards, flat-top grills, etc.

 Always use clean kitchen tools for food preparation: pots, baking sheets, utensils, cutting boards, etc.

 Prepare meals on top of barriers like cutting boards, foil, deli paper, etc.

 Remember: If a mistake is made, you must start over and remake the allergy-friendly meal

Proper Cleaning to Remove Allergens

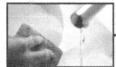
Wash with warm, soapy water

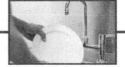
Rinse with clean water

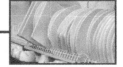
Air dry

MILK WHEAT EGGS SOY SHELLFISH PEANUTS TREE NUTS FISH SESAME

Top 9 Allergens
But over 170 foods have caused food allergy reactions

FoodAllergy.org

© FARE 2023 - 04/23

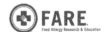
FARE
Food Allergy Research & Education

Sources of Cross-Contact

Cross-contact occurs when an allergen is unintentionally transferred from one food to another. Even a tiny amount of an allergen can cause a severe and potentially life-threatening reaction.

Source of Cross-Contact	Example:
Hands	• Handling shrimp and then preparing a salad • Touching almonds and then making pasta
Utensils, cutting boards, baking sheets, pots & pans	• Using the same spatula to flip a hamburger after a cheeseburger • Slicing cheese and then vegetables on the same cutting board
Preparation and cooking surfaces	• Preparing different kinds of sandwiches on the same countertop • Cooking fish and chicken on the same flat top grill
Steam, splatter, flour dust and crumbs	• Steam from cooking fish or shellfish touches nearby foods • Baking flour from pancake mix splatters onto bacon
Refrigerators, freezers and storage areas	• Ranch dressing drips onto a vinaigrette stored on a lower shelf • Milk leaks onto margarine stored on the same shelf
Deep fryers and cooking oils	• Making french fries in a deep fryer after chicken tenders • Reusing cooking oil to sauté green beans after sautéing fish
Condiments, nut butters and jelly/jams	• Dipping a knife used to spread peanut butter into a jelly jar • Touching the tip of a squeeze ketchup bottle to a breaded chicken breast
Shortcuts	• Picking croutons off a salad • Scraping eggs off a plate

Proper Cleaning to Remove Allergens

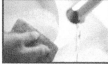

Wash with warm, soapy water

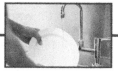

Rinse with clean water

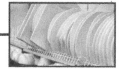

Air dry

For each new item, use clean:

Hands	Utensils	Oil and Water
Latex-free Gloves	Surfaces	Pots/Pans/Baking Sheets

 MILK   WHEAT   EGGS   SOY   SHELLFISH   PEANUTS   TREE NUTS   FISH   SESAME

Top 9 Allergens
But over 170 foods have caused food allergy reactions

FoodAllergy.org

 FARE
Food Allergy Research & Education

© FARE 2023 · 04/23

Having to do this made me absolutely mad. Like the crazy kind of mad. It was moments like those that I would think about how privileged I was to be a stay-at-home mom with the time to do this. Working moms were put in trickier positions trying to manage events at school in addition to their responsibilities at work. Neither way felt right to me. No parent should have to work harder or worry more because of how their school handled food for Field Day. I wanted the legitimate concerns around cross-contact to be taken seriously. I wanted a process put in place that kept safety at the forefront. Where there's a will there's a way.

The following year the school nurse offered to hold onto our cut up fruit in the school fridge and bring it out to my kids at the appropriate time. This was really helpful! It simplified my day tremendously and allowed me to volunteer at the event. And yet, I still wanted the school to take it more seriously. I knew my family wasn't the only family managing food allergies, but I wondered if other food allergy families were aware of the potential risks from cross-contact? Until you know, you don't know. Having her do this helped me, but it wasn't a sustainable solution.

That year the school also decided to give out popsicles at the end of the day. I had been told they stopped doing this years ago because it didn't meet the Wellness Policy, and yet they decided to "make an exception for Field Day." Believe it or not, some brands of popsicles contain milk. Good friends of ours learned this the hard way after their child had an anaphylactic reaction to a seemingly benign popsicle. What if someone grabbed the wrong box and assumed they were safe? Did the school nurse realize that popsicles could pose a threat? I didn't know and nobody had run this by me ahead of time which really bothered me. My kids weren't prepared. Shea refused to eat it because she was scared. Thomas, younger, said he didn't know what to do so he ate it. Fortunately he was fine. I continued to be a squeaky wheel, letting them know when these things happened that it wasn't ok. I felt like I was constantly sharing concerns and asking for change and it was uncomfortable. I felt like my words were falling on deaf ears and I had no idea if I was communicating in an effective way. I didn't know how to do this.

But then I was greeted with positive change. The following year two things happened. First, a letter was sent home to families asking for volunteers to send in WHOLE apples, WHOLE bananas, and WHOLE oranges or clementines for Field Day. All of these are refreshing AND allergy friendly. They present just like individually packaged snacks. I couldn't believe it! I hadn't been part of any behind the scenes discussions. I hadn't been invited to weigh in or share my thoughts. But I felt like I had earned this! I felt like this change deserved fireworks and a celebration, but it was sooo not a big deal. The school just sent the message and people just signed up and donated the food. No push back. No drama. That year I was also contacted ahead of time to review popsicle ingredients and approve them for my children. This was all so appreciated. And, it felt like a sustainable solution to safety, fun and health – which is what Field Day was all about!

ADVOCACY

Throughout much of this time, I was still wondering what on earth the policy was around managing food allergies in our schools. When I had been unable to find anything on the district website or in the handbook, I started researching like a mad woman. I was starved for useful information. What was going on at other schools? What rights did we have? I started cold calling other school nurses in different parts of the state. Sometimes they were very friendly and happily answered my questions, sometimes they forwarded me their district and school policies around food allergies, and sometimes they even shared other things they knew about food allergy management in schools. On more than one occasion, a school nurse told me they'd had a, "significantly helpful training from an allergist named Dr. Michael Pistiner" and suggested I look him up. Upon hearing this I always smiled at my end of the phone and thanked them for their help. I agreed wholeheartedly with them and was thrilled to hear he was training school nurses! Sometimes it was clear they were annoyed by my calls and questions. That was fine, I just kept going. I even called the school nurse from our previous town to confirm that Shea's classroom had been peanut-free and milk-free. It had been both. I kept all of my notes and any documents sent my way safely in a folder so I could review them as needed.

As part of my desperate attempt to learn more, and hopefully get this whole classroom allergen restriction fiasco worked out, I started learning about Massachusetts food allergy advocacy efforts. I learned that, wow, we have some real go-getters right here in the Commonwealth!

Laurel Franceour, who Jay and I had reached out to about the mislabeled guacamole, graduated from Suffolk Law School and has been a practicing lawyer since 1996.

504 Plans

504 Plans are available under a federal civil rights law, Section 504 of the Rehabilitation Act of 1973. The U.S. Department of Education (USDOE) regulation to implement Section 504 (34 C.F.R. Part 104) applies to schools and programs that receive federal money and encompasses a wide range of health conditions, including life-threatening food allergy. USDOE's Office for Civil Rights lists allergy as an example of a hidden disability for the purpose of Section 504, and further explains how a food allergy, for many children, would be considered a disability under 504. Section 504 allows you to create, in collaboration with the school, a 504 Plan, which is a written management plan outlining how the school will address the individual needs of your child, and allow your child to participate safely and equally alongside his/her peers during all normal facets of the school day. To begin the 504 process, you need to contact the school's 504 Coordinator. This could be someone who works at the school, or it could be someone who works for your school district.[24]

24. Section 504 and Written Management Plans - https://www.foodallergy.org/resources/section-504-and-written-management-plans

When her son had a life-threatening allergic reaction to eggs in kindergarten, she decided to dedicate her practice to improving the lives of people with food allergies through her advocacy and legal work. She is a national speaker on the topic of food allergy and the law. She has drafted legislation in Massachusetts and has testified at the state and federal level.[25] She is an author and speaker, has presented webinars, and has appeared in several media outlets over the years. I bought and read Laurel's book *How to Advocate for your Food Allergic Child* then gave her a call. Our conversation was disappointing simply because she didn't have an easy answer for me. However, she told me about the Massachusetts state guidelines and the CDC guidelines for managing food allergies in schools. These documents were new to me, this was big! She also asked if I had a 504 Plan in place, to which I responded that we did not. I really didn't know much about how they related to food allergies but made a note to try and learn more.

Through an online search, I found the food allergy management guidelines that the state of Massachusetts had created in 2002 on the Department of Education's website. My understanding is that we were the first state in the country to create such guidelines (go Massachusetts!) and that this document was used to pave the way for the national guidelines that later came out from the CDC. I was even more excited when I learned that Massachusetts had revisited and

25. Francoeur Law Office https://www.theallergylawyer.com/

updated guidelines in 2016. I was excited to see Dr. Pistiner's name among the experts who reviewed and contributed to the development of the guidelines. The only problem with the guidelines is that they were voluntary.

Another powerhouse in the Massachusetts food allergy advocacy community is Jan Hanson, a nationally recognized food allergy educator, speaker, and author with over 25 years experience in food allergy education. She founded her consulting company, Educating For Food Allergies, LLC, in 2001, and has authored two books and multiple articles. She is the current president of the New England Chapter of Asthma and Allergy Foundation of America (AAFA). I think it was another food allergy mom who first told me about Jan. When I saw all that she had done I couldn't wait to speak with her. I called and learned that she is also a food allergy mom and had been at this since before my kids were born. She had a lot of experience under her belt. I bought and read her book *Food Allergies: A Recipe For Success At School*, then scheduled an appointment with her. Lucky for me, her office was only 20 minutes away. I shared our story and our situation. We reviewed the state and CDC guidelines together. She validated my concerns, gave me some tips and helped boost my confidence to push on. She also mentioned that we may want to consider putting 504 Plans in place for our kids.

As an aside, in the coming years I sat with both Laurel and Jan at the State House in Boston to give testimony for food allergy legislation. I am grateful for these women and the work they have done to further awareness, education, and legislation in Massachusetts.

As I continued to learn more I started to wonder if a 504 Plan was something we should pursue. It was strange. I had learned about 504 Plans in college when I was studying to be a classroom teacher, but they had never been connected to food allergies from what I could remember. As a food allergy parent, the little I had heard about 504 Plans was negative. I had heard stories from other food allergy parents, whose children were older than mine, that schools often responded defensively to 504 requests. As though requesting and pursuing a 504 for your food allergic child was like telling the school you didn't trust them. Casually, I was advised to stay away if I wanted to keep the peace at school.

The idea of pursuing a 504 Plan didn't feel like much of a partnership to me. I was confused. Our relationship with the school was already strained so I certainly didn't want to make things worse, especially while we were waiting for a decision on the allergen designation for Shea's classroom. We decided to hold off. We didn't want to risk adding fuel to the fire. I feel it's important, as I write this all these years later, to include that I have seen a shift around this. Many families I know have pursued 504 Plans and their schools have been very professional and accommodating for the entire process. As you will read, we eventually pursued 504 Plans for both Shea and Thomas, and our schools have been great!

Fighting With the School

In the meantime, things remained challenging at school. I remember saying to friends, "we are still fighting with the school." Fighting. I couldn't believe this was a word I was using to describe the relationship we had with our children's elementary school. I tried to maintain a positive school vibe for my kids, hiding my fear and the deep disappointment I was experiencing. I wanted, no I needed, school to be a positive, happy, safe place for them and this divide often made me feel sick to my stomach. There were days I debated sending them. Shea in particular. While Thomas's classroom was free of all known allergens "because they are so young," Shea's classroom was still peanut-free, dairy-full, and she was still getting hives. Every time we got a call about hives and Benadryl, Jay and I were reminded that dairy was not managed safely in the classroom. You better believe we were documenting each incident like crazy people! Staying patient during this time was one of the hardest things I've ever had to do. I checked in with the District Nurse Leader every few weeks and she would simply respond that they didn't know yet. The waiting continued while we tried to figure out what to do next. It's easy for the me-of-today to want to go back in time and tell the me-of-yesteryear what to do (fight harder, fight louder, go over her head, go to the media), but I had never been in a situation like this. I never liked confrontation so I was already out of my comfort zone. In addition to navigating daily life with food allergies we had to learn how to navigate advocacy efforts. Jay and I thought we were doing everything right.

One day I got a call from a substitute nurse letting me know Shea was in her office with hives. She wanted to know if she should give her Benadryl. I was about 15 minutes away running an errand. I wasn't sure how bad the hives were compared to other times so I didn't know how to answer. If we could avoid Benadryl she wouldn't have to deal with getting tired. But if she needed it, I didn't want them depriving her of the relief. Frustrated and stressed, I asked if she could please text me a picture of the hives. I figured that would be easier than rushing back. She was sympathetic but told me she was not allowed to. In a moment of frustration I said something to the effect of "Ugh, ok fine. I'll make a trip back to the school yet AGAIN to check on hives yet AGAIN. It almost makes me want to get a 504 Plan in place, this has been so ridiculous. I'm sorry, it's not your fault, I'm just so tired of this." She responded that she was sorry and she understood. I headed to my car and before I even arrived at the school, she had emailed me the information to start the 504 Plan process. I couldn't believe it. Nobody from the school district had ever provided me with this information before. In fairness, I had never asked for it. I had been scared and wasn't sure what to ask for. I sure did appreciate having it handed to me. Finally someone seemed to care. Following that day, we took the necessary steps and finally put a 504 Plan in place for both kids.

It was nearly four months before we officially heard back from the District Nurse Leader about the classroom designation. They had finally made a decision (to this day I have no idea who "they" were). She informed us it would be "too much trouble for other families to have the added restriction of milk" so they decided to have the class eat snack in the cafeteria and the classroom would be food-free. She also said that students would be given a hand wipe to use before they went back to class to minimize cross-contact.

AMAZING! FANTASTIC! Literally, the best idea of all! Take all allergens out of the learning environment without inconveniencing any families. It was perfect!

And yet we wondered, why had this taken so long? Why had this been so hard? Did the sudden decision have anything to do with our request for a 504 Plan? We didn't know. All I knew was the incredible relief I felt to have this challenging and stressful experience behind us.

TO BE OR NOT TO BE DAIRY-FREE

For a while things felt under control and we knew what to expect. That was until Shea started fifth grade. This would be her final year at the elementary school. When we met for her annual 504 Plan meeting before the start of school, we learned that the school did not want an allergen ban in her classroom. We wanted the dairy-free designation in her classroom. In fourth grade her classroom was allergen-free (milk included and we didn't have to fight it), instead of having the kids eat in the cafeteria for snack time as they had for third grade. I still preferred the cafeteria option because it eliminated restrictions on other families, but my priority was her safety in the classroom and that had been provided. With this new issue on the table I could feel myself going back into the defensive mode I'd spent so much time in two years prior. Why were they doing this?

The District Nurse Leader was called back to our school to confer. She was in agreement with the school. In fact, it appeared the town was removing allergen-free classrooms for all fifth graders in the district. This was bigger than just Shea's classroom. How I wished I knew other fifth grade parents of food allergic kiddos to partner with. Even with SAFE in existence there were still plenty of families out there we hadn't connected with. The Nurse Leader argued, "we need to help kids become more independent and learn to take on more responsibility for their allergies as they prepare for middle school next year. There are no restrictions at the middle school level so their allergens can be anywhere." This might sound like an acceptable statement, but it was not to me. I still get worked up thinking back on this.

First of all, in real life, when we would go to a restaurant we would wipe down the table and chairs, the menus and ketchup bottles before we sat down to eat. When we would go on a plane we would wipe down the seats, armrests, TVs, and trays before the kids sat down. We would also have them wear pants and long sleeves. The presence of their allergens in the real world was something our kids had grown up with. They knew we would never leave the house without their epinephrine. We had trained them to take on a more active role in managing their allergies as it became more developmentally appropriate. This suggestion that the school needed to help our kids become more independent and take on more responsibility related to their allergies was insulting. We had that under control, thank you very much.

Second, and just as infuriating, I knew she was wrong. Our town had built a new Middle School two years prior. It was practically brand new. When it first opened I was invited to meet with health teachers and offer insight regarding food use and food allergies for their food labs program. I learned during this time that aside from the food lab classrooms, no food was allowed anywhere in the building outside the cafeteria. When I heard this I did a happy dance inside. One less thing to worry about. You can imagine my frustration as she sat there and told us their allergens could be anywhere. I challenged her, "How is this preparing my child for middle school when in middle school she will have less exposure to her allergen than what you are proposing for this year?" I was frustrated. Please, focus on keeping my child safe while she is here and we can deal with next year, next year. In the end they agreed to keep her primary classroom allergen-free. Advocacy means speaking up when things don't seem right. Being the voice for your child.

Get Peanuts Off the Pedestal

It is really pretty simple. Nuts are dangerous for nut allergic individuals. Milk is dangerous for milk allergic individuals. Shellfish is dangerous for shellfish allergic individuals. Sesame is dangerous for sesame allergic individuals. You get it. If someone tells you they have a food allergy, take it seriously. All food allergies need to be taken seriously.

It likely comes from managing multiple food allergies in my home, but when I see one allergen being called out over others (ahem, nuts), it doesn't sit well with me. I acknowledge that my thoughts on this are not the popular way of thinking, and plenty of people do not agree with me. But I also acknowledge that, I've had this conversation with a number of people over the years and after fully discussing it, they often get it. Believe it or not, there is a large group of people who agree with this line of thinking, you just don't hear about it a lot.

My church is a beautiful, loving, kind, and inclusive community. After Sunday morning service we go to the Parish building for coffee hour. The building houses a nursery school during the week. As you approach the door you are met by a sign, "This is a nut-free building." I believe the sign has been there for a long time. I believe it is specifically for the preschool, but since congregants of the church share the space with the preschool we are expected to abide by the rule.

To be blunt, I don't like the sign and I don't like the rule. Here's why. My children are allergic to milk. Milk is dangerous for them the same way nuts are dangerous to someone who is allergic to nuts, like Thomas. Nuts can cause anaphylaxis. So can milk. So can other allergens. Nuts can be life-threatening. So can milk. So can other allergens. As you can imagine during a coffee hour it is commonplace to have milk, creamer, cream cheese, cheese, and yogurt as examples. To be in a space where people are concerned about nuts and have an awareness of nuts, but lack the same concern and awareness with regard to other allergens, well it doesn't feel inclusive. It was just another space we had to be careful and aware. The difference was, a lot of people thought they were aware. They thought the space was welcoming and accommodating for people and families managing food allergies. Rather, they were singularly nut aware. And this made it harder for some to understand the seriousness of allergies besides nuts, like milk. Sometimes we packed safe snacks for our kids but other kids were still eating their allergens. With no awareness around hand washing, if they went out to play on the playground afterwards, we had to be aware of what they touched and remind them not to touch their face at all and wash their hands right afterward. Sometimes it was just easier to skip coffee hour and go home. Neither option felt great. Not because the kids couldn't eat most of the food (we could have brought safe food from home) but because there wasn't an awareness around the severity of their milk allergy or the importance of hand washing which would have minimized cross-contact concerns.

I started talking about the food allergies our family manage with people. More than one person I spoke with assumed my kids were allergic to nuts. "You must be happy knowing this is a nut-free building!" They weren't being malicious. They weren't being disrespectful. They just didn't understand. They hadn't been educated around this. And why would they if they didn't live it? I'm a firm believer that knowledge is power. Likewise, there is plenty I don't know about. I need to be educated so I can properly understand. Milk allergy didn't fit their preconceived notions around food allergies the way nuts did. The damn peanuts were on a pedestal. I mean, I remember talking about this with someone one Sunday, as they were eating a bagel with cream cheese while holding a cup of coffee with creamer in it. But no nuts. Don't let the nuts in.

How do we get the peanuts down?, I would wonder. My kids know I feel strongly about the importance of respecting all allergies. They have asked me about the sign over the years and I simply respond, I don't agree with it. This sign, this approach, is not unique to our church. There are nut-free schools, nut-free buildings, nut-free camps, nut-free museums, nut-free tables, nut-free sporting events, and more. It's not hard to see how they ended up on the pedestal. But, when we elevate the seriousness of one allergy we minimize the seriousness of other allergies. Let me say that again. *When we elevate the seriousness of one allergy we minimize the seriousness of other allergies.* I've debated this with people in the food allergy community.

Their perspective is that you have to start somewhere, and an awareness around nuts will trickle down to help increase awareness around other allergies. At first I conceded. Maybe they were right, as much as I didn't like it. But this has continued for years now – over a decade in my own experience. At this point I say, confidently, I do not agree. The "trickle down" has not happened. I would argue that in fact, the opposite has happened. More and more, people have been led to believe nut allergies are more dangerous than other allergies, and this is a problem.

I can't tell you how many times I have told someone my child has a milk allergy and they respond, "Oh you're so lucky it's not a nut allergy, those are very serious." They're right. Nut allergies are serious. But they are incorrectly assuming that milk isn't as serious. It falls on me to try to educate them. "Actually a milk allergy is just as serious as a nut allergy. It is different from lactose intolerance. We have to be careful." To which they reply "No, kids with nut allergies can die." And as much as I absolutely hate to do it, I say "So can kids with milk allergies." I usually get a look of shock. They're familiar with lactose intolerance but that's not life-threatening. If milk has the potential to be life-threatening why haven't they heard about it? And why do they hear about nuts so much? I imagine this is what goes through their mind. Next I usually share that both of my children are allergic to milk and one of them is also allergic to peanuts and tree nuts. Meaning, we manage the nut world and the milk world. I find that this helps get trust that I know what I'm talking about. Managing both milk and nut allergies allows me to speak to this issue. It allows me to have my strong opinion. I see very clearly that these two allergens are not respected equally, making it harder for those who navigate milk allergy.

According to the CDC, food allergy prevalence in children increased by 50% between 1997 and 2011. And a 2015-2016 survey indicates an average of 1 in 13 kids has a food allergy.[25] That's a lot of kids. There are a number of theories, but no concrete answers as to why. In the late 90s, into the early 2000s, banning nuts was what food allergy awareness looked like. Peanuts were the enemy. Get them out of lunch! Get them out of school! Lumped together with tree nut allergies, the overarching term "nuts" became commonplace. At the time there may have been an invisible badge of honor to be a "nut-free school" or have "nut-free classrooms" or "nut-free tables."

But times have changed. Nuts are not the most common food allergy. According to information from 2018

25. https://www.foodallergy.org/resources/facts-and-statistics

peanuts, milk, shellfish, and tree nuts are the most common food allergies in children.[26]

Frustrated by the sign at my church and hopeful of making positive change, I thought that with the right education and awareness people might start to agree that the sign should come down and be open to finding ways to more safely include all food allergic individuals, or anyone with a significant dietary restriction. So I reached out to and met with a committee with the church followed by a committee with the Nursery School. I think my fear and frustration were too strong. I struggled to communicate about it without emotion. While some people were receptive to my ideas, those with decision making power were not. I wasn't making the difference I had hoped to. At one point it was suggested that we could put up a new sign beside the original sign. The new sign would read "we are allergy aware." I loved the idea of this sign, but without taking down the "nut-free building" it sort of felt like an oxymoron. I believe that to be truly allergy aware we wouldn't ban allergens. Instead we would talk about ways to approach shared food that would keep everyone safely included, and maybe even keep epinephrine stored on site [Allergy Emergency Kits are an amazing option for this – allergyemergencykit.com]. With a nut ban in place we were inadvertently creating a false sense of security.

26. Gupta RS, Warren CM, Smith BM, Blumenstock JA, Jiang J, Davis MM, Nadeau KC. "The Public Health Impact of Parent-Reported Childhood Food Allergies in the United States." Pediatrics 2018; 142(6):e20181235.

Real life example of this false sense of security

An evening fundraising event was held for parents at a school that has designated themselves nut-free. One of the students was dropped off at the end to get a ride home with their parents who were helping clean up. Leftover brownies were on a table so the student grabbed one and gobbled it up. This student has a peanut allergy. They quickly realized the brownie had nuts because they started to react. The family acted quickly and fortunately their child was ok, but this can happen. It's impossible to guarantee a space will remain free of whatever banned allergen (often nuts) and potentially dangerous assumptions can be made. If there hadn't been a ban at the school, I imagine the student wouldn't have eaten the brownie without asking about it first, and this scary experience could have been avoided. Intentional or not, food can end up where it's not supposed to. Things get snuck in or people don't know certain foods are prohibited, or maybe they just forget. I suggest we address the elephant in the room and stop promoting a false sense of security with large scale bans.

I wanted our church to become a leader in the community around food allergy awareness. I spoke with our Minister about this and he said, "People need to learn. Is there a way you could help educate them?" Ok, an action item. He reminded me that "Hobby Day" was in a couple of weeks. This was a unique opportunity during coffee hour to set up a table and share about one's hobbies. Church members would be able to ask questions and look at your display. He encouraged me to participate and use the opportunity to help educate our church community. I was all in.

I had never done something like this, but I was excited and needed a plan. Keep it short and sweet, I thought. Be impactful, be memorable, give people an experience rather than a lecture. I got to thinking. Labels are very important for food allergy families, and can be confusing. Maybe it would be fun to look at labels with people and challenge them. Pages 140-141 show just a few labels currently in my kitchen show how varied labels can be.

Hand washing is also very important with food allergy management. Most people don't realize that by washing their hands after eating they can help those managing food allergies. Hand washing is important for removing food protein. A small research study found that soap and water and commercial hand wipes removed allergens but hand sanitizing gels did not.[27]

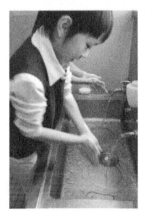

Food-Allergy-Friendly Zone!

Please wash hands before and after handling or eating food.

 Wet

 Lather

 Scrub

 Rinse

 Dry

For more information on managing food allergies, please visit **foodallergy.org**

 FARE
Food Allergy Research & Education

foodallergy.org

27. Perry, T.T. et al. "Distribution of peanut allergen in the environment." Journal of Allergy and Clinical Immunology 113.5 (2004): 973-6.

(continues p. 142)

Variations of Ingredient Labels

Vit. D (0% DV), Calcium (6% DV), Iron (6% DV), Potas. (4% DV).
INGREDIENTS: ORGANIC ALMONDS (NOT ROASTED).
CONTAINS: TREE NUTS. MAY CONTAIN: PEANUTS, OTHER TREE NUTS, MILK, SOY, WHEAT AND EGGS.
DISTRIBUTED BY FOODHOLD U.S.A., LLC, LANDOVER, MD 20785 • Certified Organic by NOFA-NY

INGREDIENTS: Enriched Flour (Wheat Flour, Niacin, Reduced Iron, Thiamine Mononitrate, Riboflavin, Folic Acid), Tapioca Malt Syrup (Tapioca Syrup, Malt Extract), Canola Oil, Salt, Maltodextrin, Modified Cornstarch, Yeast, Enzyme Modified Butterfat (Milk), Natural Flavoring, Sugar, Soda.
CONTAINS: WHEAT, MILK.

MADE FROM: ENRICHED WHEAT FLOUR (FLOUR, NIACIN, REDUCED IRON, THIAMINE MONONITRATE, RIBOFLAVIN, FOLIC ACID), SUGAR, VEGETABLE OILS (PALM, PALM KERNEL AND/OR SOYBEAN AND HYDROGENATED SOYBEAN), SEMI SWEET CHOCOLATE (SUGAR, CHOCOLATE, CHOCOLATE PROCESSED WITH ALKALI, COCOA BUTTER, MILKFAT, SOY LECITHIN, VANILLA EXTRACT), EGGS, CONTAINS 2% OR LESS OF: CORNSTARCH, SALT, BAKING SODA, SOY LECITHIN, MILKFAT, PEPPERMINT OIL, NATURAL FLAVOR, NONFAT MILK.
CONTAINS: WHEAT, MILK, SOY, EGGS.

INGREDIENTS: PURE GLUTEN FREE OATS*, CHOCOLATE* (CANE SUGAR*, UNSWEETENED CHOCOLATE*, COCOA BUTTER*), AGAVE SYRUP*, SPRINKLES* (RICE CRISPS* [RICE FLOUR*, CANE SYRUP*, SALT], VEGETABLE GLYCERIN*, SUNFLOWER OIL*, BEET POWDER* [ADDED FOR COLOR], PURPLE SWEET POTATO POWDER [ADDED FOR COLOR] [MALTODEXTRIN, PURPLE SWEET POTATO EXTRACT, CITRIC ACID], SPIRULINA EXTRACT* [ADDED FOR COLOR]), BROWN RICE SYRUP*, INVERT CANE SYRUP*, SUNFLOWER OIL*, BROWN RICE CRISPS*, GLUTEN FREE OAT FLOUR*, NATURAL FLAVOR*, VEGETABLE EXTRACTS (SPINACH, BROCCOLI, CARROTS, TOMATOES, BEETS, SHIITAKE MUSHROOMS), SALT, AGAR*. *ORGANIC.

INGREDIENTS: ENRICHED WHEAT FLOUR (FLOUR, NIACIN, REDUCED IRON, THIAMINE MONONITRATE, RIBOFLAVIN, FOLIC ACID), SUGAR, VEGETABLE OIL SHORTENING (PALM AND PALM KERNEL OILS), COCOA (PROCESSED WITH ALKALI), CARAMEL COLOR, INVERT SUGAR, SALT, BAKING SODA, SOY LECITHIN, PEPPERMINT OIL, NATURAL AND ARTIFICIAL FLAVOR.
CONTAINS: WHEAT, SOY.
MANUFACTURED IN A SHARED FACILITY WITH: MILK, PEANUTS, COCONUT.
MANUFACTURED BY: ABC BAKERS

Dedicated facility free from the following common allergens:

- Peanut
- Tree Nuts
- Dairy
- Egg
- Wheat & Gluten
- Soy
- Sesame
- Fish & Shellfish

Iron 4mg 19%
Potassium 23mg 0%

3 Net Carbs Per Serving.

ingredients: Water, OWYN™ Protein Blend (Pea Protein, Organic Pumpkin Seed Protein, Organic Flax Oil), Vegetable Fiber, Organic Cane Sugar, Sunflower Oil, Natural Flavors, Sunflower Lecithin, Guar Gum, Greens Blend (Broccoli, Spinach, Kale), Monk Fruit Extract, Himalayan Pink Salt.

Variations of Ingredient Labels

INGREDIENTS: Sweet Brown Rice Flour, Brown Rice Flour, Tapioca Starch, Arrowroot Powder, Rice Syrup Solids (Rice Syrup Solids, Rice Protein, Tocopherols), Ground Vanilla Bean,Cream of Tartar, Citrus Fiber, Baking Soda and Salt.

INGRÉDIENTS : Farine de Riz Brun Gluant, Farine de Riz Brun, Fécule de Tapioca, Arrow-root en Poudre, Solids de Sirop de Riz (Solids de Sirop de Riz, Protéine de Riz, Tocopherols), Gousse de Vanille Moulue, Crème de Tartre, Fibre d'Argrumes, Bicarbonate de Sodium et Sel.

Our facility is free from allergens listed on bottom.

Notre installation est exempte des allergènes indiqués au fond.

per serving **60** Vitamin D 0mcg 0% • Calcium 10mg 0% • Iron 0mg 0% • Potassium 70mg 0%

INGREDIENTS: CANE SUGAR, UNSWEETENED CHOCOLATE, COCOA BUTTER.
MADE IN A DEDICATED NUT AND GLUTEN FREE FACILITY. THE FACILITY ALSO PROCESSES DAIRY AND SOY; HOWEVER, THIS PRODUCT IS PRODUCED ON A DEDICATED DAIRY- AND SOY-FREE LINE. INGREDIENTS HAVE BEEN ADDITIONALLY TESTED TO ENSURE STRICT ALLERGEN CONTROL STANDARDS ARE MET.

per serving **100** Vitamin D 0% • Calcium 0% • Iron 0% • Potassium 0%

Ingredients: Organic Soybean Oil, Water, Organic Egg Yolk, Organic Distilled Vinegar, Contains less than 2% of each: Salt, Organic Cane Sugar, Organic Mustard Seed, Organic Lemon Juice Concentrate, Organic Natural Flavor, Organic Oleoresin Paprika (for color).

Ⓐ ALLERGENS: Contains Eggs.

Distributed By Wegmans Food Markets, Inc. Rochester, NY 14603

INGREDIENTS: UNBLEACHED ENRICHED FLOUR (WHEAT FLOUR, NIACIN, REDUCED IRON, THIAMINE MONONITRATE (VITAMIN B1), RIBOFLAVIN (VITAMIN B2), FOLIC ACID), SEMISWEET CHOCOLATE CHIPS (SUGAR, CHOCOLATE, COCOA BUTTER, DEXTROSE, MILK, SOY LECITHIN), SUGAR, SOYBEAN AND/OR CANOLA OIL, PALM OIL, HIGH FRUCTOSE CORN SYRUP, LEAVENING (BAKING SODA, AMMONIUM PHOSPHATE), SALT, NATURAL AND ARTIFICIAL FLAVOR, CARAMEL COLOR.

CONTAINS: WHEAT, MILK, SOY.

INGREDIENTS: CANE SUGAR, COCOA (PROCESSED WITH ALKALI), TAPIOCA STARCH, RICE FLOUR, BAKING POWDER (SODIUM ACID PYROPHOSPHATE, BAKING SODA, CORN STARCH, MONOCALCIUM PHOSPHATE), SALT, NATURAL VANILLA FLAVOR.

DISTRIBUTED BY
KING ARTHUR BAKING COMPANY, INC.
NORWICH, VERMONT 05055
800-827-6836 | KingArthurBaking.com

NON-DAIRY*

Certified Gluten-Free by GFCO | GFCO.org

For information on allergens and cross-contact prevention, visit: KingArthurBaking.com/allergen-program

Our products are free from:
Nos produits ne contiennent :

☑ wheat / blé   ☑ mustard / moutarde
☑ gluten / gluten   ☑ sulfites / sulfites
☑ egg / oeuf   ☑ sesame / sésame
☑ dairy / produit laitier   ☑ caseine / caséine
☑ peanuts / arachides   ☑ fish / poisson
☑ tree nuts / noix   ☑ crustaceans / crustacé
☑ soy / soya   ☑ shellfish / mollusques

TESTED FOR TOP 8 ALLERGENS.

OWYN's ingredients and finished products are independently tested for detection of the top 8 allergens every lot, every time.

Increasing Hand Washing in Schools

I remember talking to the school about hand washing. How it is an important element in keeping kids with food allergies safe. I remember they told us they couldn't enforce it. This surprised me since hand washing is just good hygiene for kids and germs, but also because it could help keep our kids and others with food allergies safer. It got me thinking about my teaching days. One sink in the classroom and potentially 22 sets of hands to wash? From a time perspective alone, that would have been a nightmare. When they all wanted a drink from the water fountain after gym, it took 15 minutes. But I'm a big believer that where there's a will, there's a way. Was there a way to increase hand washing in an easy way that would make sense in a school setting? Then it came to me. Trough sinks. What if the cafeteria and possibly other areas in the building were lined with trough sinks that could allow 10 or so kids to wash their hands at the same time? Foot pedals so their hands wouldn't be needed, and multiple spouts so they could spread out. I would love to know if there are schools out there with something like this in use. I have yet to see this sort of thing in action in a school, but maybe someday! Something to consider with new school building plans.

Lastly, I thought about epinephrine auto-injectors (refer back to page 19 for details) and how they come with trainers for practicing. How cool would it be to let people see them and try the trainers out?! I narrowed my ideas down to these three areas of awareness and education that I thought were beneficial for other people to learn about.

Hobby Day went well. People seemed interested and I enjoyed it. I felt like I could do even more. Something to reach more people. When SAFE had the opportunity to apply for a COA (Community Outreach Award) with FARE that year, I proposed a larger event at my church around awareness and education. My minister was supportive of this idea. Lauren and I expanded on the plan I had used for Hobby Day. We wanted to provide people with experiences that could help them learn so we included a label reading station, a hand washing station and an epi trainer station. I wanted to add an educational component too so I contacted Dr. Pistiner and invited him to come as a guest speaker. He was in! The event would be two parts. Dr. Pistiner's presentation for the first half, followed by stations to explore for the second half. We opened the event to my church community as well as the public and advertised it via social media, newspaper, flyers, and email. I hoped that people with a connection to our church or to the preschool would join us to learn more.

We had a great showing. Few of the attendees were members of my church and I don't know if any families from the preschool came. I had mixed emotions about this. While I had hoped to further educate my church community, on the whole, it was a success! People had joined us to listen and learn. Many kids and parents from SAFE had volunteered to help, which was terrific. I was proud of what we had provided the community and I hoped that in time, through continued awareness efforts, we could influence change. In the meantime we were expanding awareness in the larger community, which was awesome.

I watched for additional opportunities to keep educating. I was able to partner with the Director of Religious Education to find more ways to do this. One year we coordinated a pumpkin painting event with the option to do teal pumpkins.

Teal Pumpkin Project

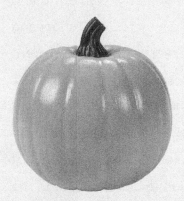

The Teal Pumpkin Project is a simple way to make trick-or-treating safer and more inclusive for the one in 13 children living with food allergies, and many others impacted by intolerances and other conditions. Placing a teal pumpkin on your doorstep signals that, in addition to candy, you offer non-food trinkets and treats that are safe for all trick or treaters. Thanks to Becky Basalone, a mother-of-two and the creator of the Teal Pumpkin Project, Halloween is getting more teal and far less spooky for children with food allergies. It was in the fall of 2012 that Basalone, the director of a local Tennessee food allergy support group, first had the bright idea of painting a pumpkin teal, the color of food allergy awareness, and handing out non-food items. What she didn't know was that her teal pumpkin would become a nationwide symbol for Halloween food allergy awareness. In fact, it's even taking off in Canada and Britain.[28]

28. Origin of the Teal Pumpkin Project - Interview with Becky Basalone - https://www.allergicliving.com/2014/10/23/the-origin-of-the-teal-pumpkin-project-interview-with-becky-basalone-facet/

We also coordinated safe food for movie nights and game nights that were hosted by the church. This was really helpful and allowed my family to more easily participate in these events. It was also helping to increase awareness among other families. Coffee Hour, which followed Sunday service, started to include allergy friendly, pre-packaged options for my children and anyone else who needed them. I was invited to do a short food allergy awareness lesson with our youth at the start of each church year.

Success doesn't always look the way we expect. While the sign on the door still stares back at us each time we enter the building, progress of other kinds has been made. There is increased awareness and my children have been safely included in much of the programming. All of that is absolutely worth celebrating. Is there still room for improvement? There is, but it's all part of the journey. For now, we celebrate the progress that has been made, and I hope that in time peanuts (and other nuts) will lose their coveted position on the pedestal.

Food Allergy 411

"The beautiful thing about learning is nobody can take it away from you." ~B.B. King

As Chief Operating Officer of my food allergy family, I worried. A lot. Probably an unhealthy amount. If *we* struggled to keep our kids safe, how could we expect others to keep them safe? Awareness and education. That's what came to mind.

At the time of Shea's anaphylactic reaction at my Dad's wedding we were living in a wonderful, family-friendly neighborhood. The kids often bounced from house to house, yard to yard playing together. This was new to us, and as happy as I was, I was also nervous. Today my kids self-carry their epinephrine auto-injectors when they go out, but back then I carried them. So, what to do when they went out without me? One of the things I worried about was if another mom kindly offered snacks to the kids that weren't safe and my kids got confused and accepted something, then reacted, and the mom wasn't prepared to help them. My kids were young enough that I didn't feel completely confident they would know what to do. Fortunately, we hadn't been tested. Up to this point they had always been in the direct care of someone who knew about their allergies. I wanted to encourage their independence but I also needed to ensure their safety.

I had an idea. Most moms I knew enjoyed a night out. Ladies' Nights, Book Clubs, whatever the reason, so I decided to host a night at my house with some of the neighborhood moms. But this Ladies' Night would have a twist. The invitation said something like "Come for a fun night with wine, apps, desserts... and a side of food allergy info." I was looking for a comfortable and appropriate opportunity to be open, honest, and direct with them. To tell them what my kids were allergic to, what that meant, and how they could help me keep them safe. I also wanted to answer any questions they might have. I had no idea what their own food allergy experiences were. I called it "Food Allergy 411."

If you build it they will come! It was wonderful. Not only was it fun to have a ladies' night, but when the time came to talk about allergies, they were a really captive audience. They listened, they asked questions. I felt much better being able to explain things, and they seemed to appreciate the opportunity. We practiced with epi trainers so they could see what they looked like and try them out first hand. We also used a real, expired, epinephrine auto-injector on an orange to get a better sense of how much force is needed to activate the needle.

I was grateful to each of them for taking the time to come. For a few years I made it an annual event. I'd invite new families who came into our lives, and sometimes friends would bring someone along who they thought might benefit. One of my friends who is also a classroom teacher said, "This was great. I learned a lot and I feel like I understand food allergies better." Yay! Mission accomplished. That's how I felt after attending the workshop at Boston Children's Hospital. As a former teacher myself, I had failed to recognize my own child's anaphylaxis even though I had been trained. The training I received was more about *how* to use an epinephrine auto-injector and less about understanding *when* to use one. I was happy to help these women better understand food allergies, and it was icing on the cake if I could help teachers.

The feedback was positive. I was introduced to someone a few years ago, and when I told her where I lived she said "I have a friend who lives over there. Wait, are you the one who does those food allergy nights?! She told me all about them and it sounds great!" I laughed out loud and it certainly warmed my heart to hear this. Education and awareness. Facts over fear. I can't think of a better way. It would be fun to "take this show on the road" so to speak. Certification exists for people who want to be "Asthma Educators," but I have found no such training or certification for "Food Allergy Educators," quite unfortunately. I am compassionate towards those who have not learned about food allergies. Everything I now know came from needing to keep my children safe. I didn't learn about it when I brought my babies home from the hospital. I didn't learn about food allergies at PTO meetings or

Open House nights at school (hmm, opportunities maybe?). I learned it because I live it. I want to support those who are interested in learning more, by sharing what my family has learned.

When my kids were little I was clueless about statistics and totally afraid of social media. Online support groups probably existed, but I didn't know about them. Moms may have been coming together and connecting over their food allergy experiences, but I was unaware. I was lonely. Most of the moms I knew didn't understand what it was like, which wasn't their fault. And other kids didn't understand what my kids went through.

I have since discovered a number of Facebook groups for allergy moms/caregivers. Some groups have tens of thousands of members, some have far less. Some are specific to location, or allergen, and some aren't specific to anything other than food allergies. Groups are not created equal and there are drastically different vibes out there. I think it's important to find vibes and groups that work for you. I can search past posts to see if there is useful information when I have a question. I'm free to be a silent observer. I know to take some things with a grain of salt, but I also appreciate the insights, perspectives, and ideas of those who get it. Some groups have helped me feel less alone and reminded me that my kids aren't alone either.

Of course there are also support groups. Back when I first tried to find a support group, the closest one was on

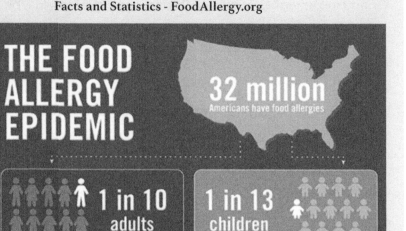

Facts and Statistics - FoodAllergy.org

THE FOOD ALLERGY EPIDEMIC

32 million Americans have food allergies

1 in 10 adults

1 in 13 children

51% More than half of adults with food allergies have experienced a severe reaction.

42% More than 40 percent of children with food allergies have experienced a severe reaction.

Some Food Allergy Facts and Statistics:

1. Results from a 2015-2016 survey of more than 38,000 children indicate that 5.6 million children, or nearly 8%, have food allergies.[29,30] That's one in 13 children, or roughly two in every classroom.

2. More than 40 percent of children with food allergies have experienced a severe allergic reaction such as anaphylaxis.[30]

3. About 40 percent of children with food allergies have multiple food allergies (more than one food to which they're allergic).[30]

4. Individuals with food allergies who also have asthma may be at increased risk for severe or fatal food allergy reactions.[31]

5. Compared to children who do not have a medical condition, children with food allergy are twice as likely to be bullied.[32]

6. Every three minutes, a food allergy reaction sends someone to the emergency room.[33]

7. Even trace amounts of a food allergen can cause a reaction.[34,35,36,37,38,39]

29. United States Census Bureau Quick Facts (2015 and 2016 estimates).

30. Gupta RS, Warren CM, Smith BM, Blumenstock JA, Jiang J, Davis MM, Nadeau KC. "The Public Health Impact of Parent-Reported Childhood Food Allergies in the United States." Pediatrics 2018; 142(6):e20181235.

31. Bock SA, Muñoz-Furlong A, Sampson HA. "Further fatalities caused by anaphylactic reactions to food, 2001–2006." J Allergy Clin Immunol. 2007; 119(4):1016-1018.

32. Herbert L, Shemesh E, Bender B. "Clinical management of psychosocial concerns related to food allergy." J Allergy Clin Immunol Pract. 2016; 4(2):205-213.

33. Clark S, Espinola J, Rudders SA, Banerji, A, Camargo CA. "Frequency of US emergency department visits for food-related acute allergic reactions." J Allergy Clin Immunol. 2011; 127(3):682-683.

34. Hefle SL, Taylor SL. "Allergenicity of edible oils." Food Technol. 1999; 53:62-70.

35. Laoprasert N, Wallen ND, Jones RT, Hefle SL, Taylor SL, Yunginger JW. "Anaphylaxis in a milk-allergic child following ingestion of lemon sorbet containing trace quantities of milk." J Food Prot. 1998; 61:1522-1524.

36. Gern JE, Yang E, Evrard HM, Sampson HA. "Allergic reactions to milk-contaminated nondairy products." N Engl J Med. 1991; 324:976-979.

37. Yunginger JW, Gauerke MB, Jones RT, Dahlberg MJE, Ackerman SJ. "Use of radioimmunoassay to determine the nature, quantity and source of allergenic contamination of sunflower butter." J Food Prot. 1983; 46:625-628.

38. Jones R, Squillace D, Yunginger J. "Anaphylaxis in a milk-allergic child after ingestion of milk contaminated kosher-pareve-labeled "dairy-free" dessert." Ann Allergy. 1992; 68:223-227.

39. Hourihane J, Kilbrun S, Nordlee J, et al. "An evaluation of the sensitivity of subjects with peanut allergy to very low doses of peanut: a randomized, double-blind, placebo-controlled food challenge study." J Allergy Clin Immunol. 1997; 100:596-600.

Martha's Vineyard, which is an island. This would have meant driving to Cape Cod (about 45 minutes) and taking about an hour-long ferry to the island. It's a beautiful spot to visit but it wasn't going to work for me to regularly attend support group meetings there. While I was disappointed, the lack of a feasible support group got me thinking about and imagining what I would want out of a support group when I found one. I imagined what people would talk about at meetings, and if there would be snacks or if that wasn't smart because, yeah, food allergies. I imagined how often support groups would probably meet. I thought about what a flyer would say if I found one. It's funny how things work out. All of those thoughts fed the process when Meghan C. and I started SAFE.

When you start talking to people about food allergies you often get a lot of the same questions: Do food allergies run in your family? Why are there so many more food allergies now than there used to be?

Between myself and Jay, none of our parents have food allergies, none of our siblings have food allergies, and none of our nieces or nephews have food allergies. I don't know how our children came to have food allergies. I don't know why multiple siblings have allergies in some families and only one in others. I don't know why so many people assume there's a genetic component.

The increase in food allergies since my own childhood is undeniable. I have two cousins who were diagnosed with food allergies when they were young, but I was just about a teenager by that time. Nobody in my class growing up, or even in our school. My grandma would often ask, "Do the kids still have those food allergies Meghan?" And I'd reply, "Yes, unfortunately they do." And in her ever optimistic way she'd ask, "Do they think they'll grow out of them?" The doctors used to say to me that plenty of kids outgrew food allergies before age five. For a long time I said, "We hope so!" but as we celebrated sixth and seventh birthdays I lost any hope of it. My reply became, "Probably not." She had ten kids and none of them had food allergies. She couldn't understand how both of my kids had food allergies. I would have loved to know why, but I didn't have the answer then and I still don't today. I have my theories. I'm sure we all do. For one thing, I have concerns around what's been done to our food over the years. I really enjoyed reading Robyn O'Brien's book, *The Unhealthy Truth*. She's been called the Erin Brokovich of the food industry. Robyn started her deep dive after her fourth child was diagnosed with food allergies. Her TedTalk is a great place to start. A lot of us in the food allergy community have more questions than answers, like *why*? *how*?

Description of *The Unhealthy Truth*

Robyn O'Brien is not the most likely candidate for an anti-establishment crusade. A Houston native from a conservative family, this MBA and married mother of four was not someone who gave much thought to misguided government agencies and chemicals in our food – until the day her youngest daughter had a violent allergic reaction to eggs, and everything changed. *The Unhealthy Truth* is both the story of how one brave woman chose to take on the system and a call to action that shows how each of us can do our part and keep our own families safe.

O'Brien turns to accredited research conducted in Europe that confirms the toxicity of America's food supply, and traces the relationship between Big Food and Big Money that has ensured that the United States is one of the only developed countries in the world to allow hidden toxins in our food – toxins that can be blamed for the alarming recent increases in allergies, ADHD, cancer, and asthma among our children. Featuring recipes and an action plan for weaning your family off dangerous chemicals one step at a time, *The Unhealthy Truth* is a must-read for every parent – and for every concerned citizen – in America today.

For now, we manage. We make safe choices and try to increase awareness. An important part of awareness for me is educating people that all food allergies need to be taken seriously. Do we need nut bans? Can we rethink food use and designate food-free areas? Can food spaces have systems in place to maintain a safe environment for anyone with a food allergy? I believe this is all possible if we start with our young people and we are consistent. Let's create new norms. Let's teach people how to safely eat together. Hand washing and proper cleaning protocols are important. Having access to public sinks would be helpful along with ensuring those who clean eating areas are trained properly. Greater precautions are needed with young children until they learn how to eat safely together. It's just like the preschool approach my cousin's wife Danielle told me about. Where there's a will there's a way and education is a friendly avenue for encouraging the "will."

Making It Official

As you will recall, following my first Healthy Elementary Schools Task Force Meeting, another mom volunteered to go school to school with me promoting the Party in a Bag idea. I will never forget her kindness and support. It was a neat experience to connect with nearly all of the elementary school principals, as well as most of the school nurses. One principal in particular was especially kind, open minded, and willing to hear what I had to say. While she wasn't able to get her school to make a full transition to the idea, she did share it and was supportive of my efforts.

Within a few years her role shifted to Assistant Superintendent. After one classroom party in particular, I was feeling especially frustrated. I'd had a run-in with another parent and I knew there had to be a better way. I was lost and intimidated. This shouldn't be personal. I really needed clarification on the district's policies around food allergies. I figured it would give me leverage. I had not found anything in my search, and I had spent a significant amount of time researching and learning about policies and practices of other school districts in our state. Enough was enough, I needed answers from our school district. I thought she would know where to direct me. As in the past, she was kind and helpful. She told me "This is something the district needs to work on. Will you come to the next School Committee meeting and ask about it?" Of course I would.

It turns out there had been no food allergy policy. Not in the school, not in the district. I'd been on a wild goose chase on and off for over a year.

I marked my calendar for the next School Committee meeting and made my way there, with butterflies in my stomach. I didn't typically attend School Committee meetings and certainly had never spoken up during one. I wasn't sure what to expect. Fortunately, when I walked in I saw an empty seat next to my friend Janice. Janice told me she loved School Committee meetings! She enjoyed attending, listening, and learning. In fact, she was later elected as a School Committee member. She was happy to see me there and very encouraging. When the appropriate time came, and after a little elbow nudge from her, I raised my hand and asked if there were plans to create a Life-Threatening Food Allergy Policy for the District. They spoke among themselves for a minute, then the Superintendent said he'd like to create a sub-committee to work on this. He turned his attention back to me and said, "I hope you will be part of the sub-committee." Of course! I was very excited, but also nervous and intimidated.

I had done a great deal of research by this point, reaching out to more than a dozen school districts in

Massachusetts to better understand what was happening in other parts of the state. It helped, but unfortunately, I hadn't found a model example. I wasn't seeing what I wanted to see as common practice. My ideas were out of the ordinary. I wanted learning spaces to be food-free and classroom celebrations to discontinue shared food. To many, I was a "fun killer."

This work was lonely and I wasn't sure what I was doing. Staying focused on trying to do better gave me a purpose and a way to channel some of my frustration. How could I help my family or any other families if I sat at home sulking? Unless I planned on pulling my kids out of school to homeschool them (which I did not) I had work to do. I wanted to trust that my kids, and all kids with food allergies, were safely included at school.

At the first meeting the district provided all members of the sub-committee with a document to guide our work. Because of all the research I had done in recent years, I knew what I was looking at. It was the 2002 Massachusetts state guidelines for managing food allergies in schools. You might remember me saying that our fabulous state had not only been the first to create such guidelines, but they had also reviewed and updated the guidelines in 2016. It was 2018, so why were we looking at the 2002 version? I asked. I imagined a response of, "Thank you for bringing that to our attention. We will get everyone an updated document to work from moving forward." Oh, me and my imagination.

I'm not sure why, but instead of appreciating this detail about an updated document, my question seemed to frustrate the District Nurse Leader. She asked where the newer version was, so I told her, but at the next meeting she said she couldn't find it so we wouldn't use it. I again told her where it could be found. This time she responded that if it wasn't on the Department of Elementary and Secondary Education (DESE) website we couldn't use it. I couldn't figure out why this was something to debate. The state had gone to the trouble of updating this resource. We should be using it. I reached out to DESE and it took a few weeks but they confirmed my suspicion. "We are having trouble with our website and cannot get the guidelines on it for the time being, *but we still want all schools to use the updated version.*" But it was too late, we were already crafting a policy based on the old guidelines.

Having been invited to be part of this sub-committee, I didn't want to get kicked out. Could that even happen?? I wasn't sure, but I didn't want to find out the hard way. I could see the headlines already, "Local mom kicked off sub-committee for giving District Nurse Leader a hard time." I let it go and tried to get over the fact that we were working with an outdated document. I could refer to the new guidelines as it went, when it made sense. Even if it was uncomfortable to be "just" a food allergy mom, I had the same goal as everyone else: work as a team and get a life-threatening food allergy policy in place for the school district.

Not gonna lie, I wished I had more credibility. In my research I had come across someone who was a certified asthma educator. As such, she was able to educate people about asthma. She didn't have a medical background, but this certification opened doors for her. She promoted awareness, she educated, and she was taken seriously. That's what I needed. That's what I wanted. I had determined I wanted to become a certified food allergy educator (cue the singing angels, parting clouds, and bright sunshine).

I researched how to get this type of certification. I looked. I searched. I reviewed things that caught my attention, but, ultimately, what I was looking for did not exist. It took me nearly two years to accept this. I didn't see an obvious route to being more credible. Would doors ever open for me? Would I be able to educate? Dr. Pistiner was one of the only people I knew who was educating in a way that resonated with me. The problem of course – I am not a medical professional and I wasn't about to go to Medical School. I wasn't sure what was "allowed" for someone like me.

As I thought about it I realized I did know people who were educating about food allergies. Jan Hanson was educating, but I knew she had a degree in Higher Education, which I do not have. Kyle Dine was educating too. As far as I knew he didn't have a medical background or special certification, but he was making a huge difference with awareness and education in North America! If you aren't familiar with Kyle Dine, he is an internationally known performer, educator, songwriter, speaker, and entrepreneur who works to increase awareness, inclusion, understanding, and empathy around food allergies. He has performed at more than 900 schools for over one million students!!! And, he's still going strong! From his website, "Kyle Dine performs food allergy awareness assemblies for elementary schools across North America. His brand of fun and educational performances uses music, puppets, and games to engage audiences with age-appropriate content. He has released two CDs and an educational DVD which was funded through Kickstarter. He is a keynote speaker and is the founder and CEO of Equal Eats – a company providing professional dietary cards." [www.kyledine.com] In other words, he is a rockstar in the food allergy world! Especially with kids. Kyle manages food allergies himself, so he understands this way of life. I've met him a number of times over the years at different events and conferences. So I called him.

I was curious about his take on this challenge of what's "allowed" for educators who aren't medical. He simply said to me, "I stay in my lane, Meghan. For instance, I do not talk about when to use epinephrine, I just talk about the fact that epinephrine is our friend." It totally made sense. I started thinking about how I could educate and touch on anaphylaxis without going out of my lane. I wanted my lane to include preventing allergic reactions AND knowing what to do if a reaction occurs. Without being an official Food Allergy Educator, I deferred to my inner Food Allergy Educator. I imagined what my approach would look like. While I still felt like "just" a food allergy mom, I used this shift in mindset to increase my confidence. I had a seat at the table for the policy work and I was capable of staying in my lane and helping to make a difference.

The sub-committee continued to meet and make adjustments to the documents. Around the same time an email came through from one of the room parents about a big "End of Year Ice Cream Party!" You know the emoji with the head tipped down and the hand over the forehead. Yeah, that was me. *Come on*, I thought. How does an email like this even come to be? Shea's classroom was milk-free so how on earth was an ice cream party allowed? In addition to her being excluded it also posed a safety concern due to contact reactions and accidental exposure. Ice cream is hard

---

Universal Messages

There are things I wish other people knew about food allergies. As a self-proclaimed Food Allergy Educator, I call them "Universal Messages." I wanted to narrow down the most important messages to communicate about food allergies, particularly for those who do not have or manage food allergies. I looked at resources from a number of food allergy organizations and realized they were saying many of the same things, just in different ways. I landed on five things that seemed consistent, important, and worth highlighting.

1. Take all allergies seriously.

2. Wash hands after eating.

3. Know how to help if someone has a reaction.

4. Remember kindness and prevent bullying.

5. Don't share food.

for us, always has been. It's sticky and gets everywhere. Even when safe ice cream is provided, like coconut milk ice cream, focused attention is required to prevent accidental confusion of spoons. The email took me by surprise. It distracted me mentally and emotionally. I hadn't planned on spending time figuring this out, but, here I was, yet again, pausing what I was doing to figure out some food drama at school. We needed a policy already.

The school nurse and I already had a strained relationship. I figured if I reached out to her she'd tell me something about how it's a tradition or a special occasion or something else, and I'd just have to push back. Due to our history, I didn't believe she could help me. Makes me sad to think about now. Instead I decided to go right to the source and call the mom who had sent the email. Maybe there had been some confusion that we could easily sort out. Italian ice for all the kids would be a safe option. So, I gave her a call. I expected her to say something like "Oh, I'm sorry, I didn't realize. Thanks for reaching out." I'd offer to help and she'd say, "Let's come up with a plan that works and is safe for all the kids." It was this pleasant, imaginary conversation that gave me the guts to make the call. Advocating for my kids has pushed me out of my comfort zone time and again.

But, boy, was I wrong. Not only did she NOT say any of those things, she actually asked me, "How could I do this to the other kids? Why should they be punished because of your child's food allergy?"

I wasn't prepared for this response at all. I didn't know where to begin without getting very defensive, or bursting into tears. I tried to calmly let her know that this is a life-threatening allergy and that an ice cream party both excluded and was unsafe for my daughter. She then told me about her daughter's lactose intolerance and how "sometimes it's so bad it's practically life-threatening." I feel for her child, I'm sure that can be very difficult. But we aren't talking about apples and apples when we compare food allergies and intolerances. This is a common and unfortunate misconception that folks managing food allergies often know all too well. One is life-threatening, one is not. I was done. I wasn't about to battle with a fellow mom over whose child had it worse. It had been a mistake to call her and I needed to get off the phone. I thanked her for her time and said goodbye.

But what was I supposed to do? Who were my allies? How was I supposed to keep my child safe without going crazy in the process? I was batting zero. I didn't have a great relationship with the school nurse or the district nurse, and now I had developed unhealthy relationships with some of the room parents. As I sat, an ally came to mind – the Chair of Health and Wellness for the school district. For years I had been attending his Healthy School Task Force meetings and after SAFE was founded I had been added to the agenda each month for an opportunity to share any updates from the food allergy community in town. He had come to understand some of the challenges that existed. I felt like he was one of my only allies inside the school district and I wanted to gauge if I was way off base about the ice cream party or if there was merit to my concern. He listened and said that an ice cream party didn't sound appropriate to him, but he wasn't able to do anything about it, so he suggested I contact the District Nurse Leader. It was a good suggestion but my nerves were on edge. She and I had a number of difficult interactions under our belt, and things had really been charged and challenging in recent years. But I called her and explained the situation. You know what? She was like a dog with a bone! She was infuriated that a parent was trying to do an ice cream party, because it broke the Wellness Policy. Fine, I'll take it if that's what motivates her. I just needed help and she was willing to help. She got involved and put the kibosh down on the ice cream party. Fantastic!

I was anxious for a district policy to go into effect so hopefully these types of situations would be eliminated. Having the Wellness Policy bail us out this time was great, but it wasn't sustainable from a food allergy management perspective.

The work continued. We were creating the district's first food allergy policy and procedures. While it was hard to believe, it was exciting to be part of. I was pleased to see some great ideas coming into play. During one discussion I brought up the challenges of classroom parties. The District Nurse Leader commented that party days were incredibly challenging for all the school nurses as well, being bombarded with food labels to review and questions from parents and teachers.

It was nice to be in agreement and see that neither of us were big fans of the food at parties. Her comment wasn't specific to the Wellness Policy either which gave me hope.

There were two bullet points in the document that I found most exciting. "Classroom celebrations will be food-free and can focus on fun activities." And "Classrooms will be free of known allergens." These were huge, particularly after my family's experiences. The celebration piece indicated a shift from focusing on food to focusing on fun – I loved it! The allergen-free classrooms gave schools the choice to restrict all known allergens from a classroom, or, like they had done with Shea's class, lift any restrictions and move snack time to another location. It also prioritized classrooms as learning spaces and eliminated food allergy distractions for kids who had been impacted previously. I was giddy with excitement over the progress the sub-committee was making on these documents.

Finally the day came when we had a completed draft and the School Committee was notified. The next step was for them to vote on whether or not to accept the policy and procedures. It was June. I was in North Carolina visiting Dana (Remember my friend Dana? Among other things she had taken care of Shea the day Thomas reacted to peanut butter.) the day I got the email with the date for the next School Committee meeting at which they would review the documents. This work had been such a long time coming. Dana was well aware of our food allergy journey and understood how important this was to me. I was nervous and excited, just like at the beginning.

The morning of the School Committee meeting, all sub-committee members received an email from the District Nurse Leader with an updated version of the policy and procedures documents. *Nothing like the last minute*, I thought, quickly reviewing the documents to see what updates had been made. I was shocked. The statements I had been most excited about had both been removed. I felt like I'd been punched in the gut. Like the wind had been knocked out of me. I was devastated. Apparently, there was concern that those two lines would cause pushback from School Committee members, threatening the whole thing. It was argued that to preserve overall progress this was the "best plan." I begged to differ, but I didn't have the power to change this decision.

These changes to the document left gaps in food allergy management at school that could still make things challenging for food allergy families. I knew about these gaps from personal experience. I had hoped for something better from a policy perspective but I was grateful we had 504 Plans in place because they at least gave us the opportunity to have these conversations each year. Asking for accommodations is never a guarantee but at least we *could* ask that a classroom be free of our child's allergens. We *could* ask that food not be eaten in the classroom. We *could* ask that parties not include shared food.

I knew it was important to have a policy in place but I felt like we had missed an opportunity to do something even more amazing. I had hoped we would become a model school district for others to follow. Had these statements been included they would have been an exception at the time. Other school districts weren't doing that from what I had seen, and I was so excited for us to pave a new way, to show others how it could be done. I was bummed. The School Committee voted on and accepted the Policy and Procedures documents.

I think some of my frustration came from being a big picture thinker. I didn't want my family or anyone else's to have to rely on a 504 Plan. I wanted our schools to operate in a way that ensured best practices for all children. To operate in a way that prioritized safe inclusion regardless of disability. I wanted to leave something in my wake to help the families that were coming up behind me. With a 504 Plan, kids are still "different." If their class has to approach snack time in a different way because of an accommodation in their plan, other kids might talk about it. Do 504 Plans work and keep kids safe? Yes. But do they prioritize safe inclusion? I'm not as sure. I think safe inclusion is best coming from an overarching approach. From systemic decisions. Something like a district wide policy.

As a big picture thinker I have a history of wanting big results. I don't always get them, but that's what keeps me motivated. I have had to learn, "not to let perfect be the enemy of good." I first heard this from Robyn O'Brien and was struck by it immediately. The strive for perfection can be a blessing and a curse. It overwhelms me at times, getting in the way and stunting progress, but it also keeps me wanting more, wanting better. If you manage to help make progress, consciously stop and appreciate it. It wasn't quite what I wanted, but this was progress. Our school district had a life-threatening food allergy policy in place. Finally!

Where There's a Will There's a Way

"We do not 'do' inclusion 'for' people with disabilities. Rather, it is incumbent upon us to figure out how all the things we do can be inclusive." ~Lisa Friedman

Increasing opportunities for the safe inclusion of food allergic children was consistently on my mind. Sports programs and scouting programs for example. A major challenge is that people in leadership positions for these programs are usually volunteers. Community programs rely on the generous time commitment and dedication of volunteers. It is hard to ask more of our volunteers without burning them out. Volunteers are the magic of a strong community. They are critical to additional programming for our kids. I have great respect for volunteers. And I believe where there's a will there's a way. If something was valued and prioritized by organizations could it, in time, become the norm? Was there an easy, approachable, respectful way to educate volunteers with an end goal of increasing the safe inclusion of food allergic kids in their programs? Not that I knew of, but I believed that if we could find a way, life outside the home would be easier for my family and other families who manage food allergies.

I remember when my kids played baseball and softball. It wasn't unusual for parents to bring a treat for the team after the game. This was hard for us. Sometimes one parent oversaw treats, and I could try to touch base early in the season about our allergies. But team snacks weren't always organized. Sometimes they were just for fun. I didn't always know when it would happen so I wasn't always prepared (though I did start keeping a stash), and never knew what it was going to be. Let's say I pulled out pretzels from my stash but the rest of the team was eating ice cream bars – it didn't quite cut it. I always felt like a bad mom and I always felt bad for my kids when this sort of thing happened. If other parents noticed they were genuinely apologetic, but it didn't help in the moment. There was no plan to prevent it from happening in the future and that was the part that bothered me the most. I longed for a system that worked well. Being in a town with four elementary schools meant kids from each school were mixed among the teams. This meant I didn't know all the families. I wasn't a fan of the "Hi, I'm Meghan. Can I please tell you what to do when it comes to providing snacks for team sports?" Um, no thanks! It seemed like this was something that should be mandated from above, at the organizational level, not team by team, not coach by coach, not parent by parent. The judgment piece comes in again when things like this come from the parents. At least, that's how I felt. What are best practices for the safe inclusion of kids who want to participate? This doesn't just mean food allergies, as there are other disabilities and things that can impact an individual's involvement in a group activity. How do we make sure our programs are prepared to safely include them? How do we do this systematically? That's what I want to know. That's what I want to support.

I remember hearing from a few other food allergy moms in my support group that they didn't sign their kids up for activities because of the food. It broke my heart to think of kids missing out. And yet, I understood. It is a loaded experience to participate in activities where food isn't carefully planned. On the occasions when Jay or I have signed up to coach we were able to communicate clearly with our team and limit what was shared, but we didn't want to *have to* coach. Agreeing to coach felt like a consequence rather than a choice, but it gave us an increased confidence that the kids would be safely included in all things team related. Let me be clear, NOBODY ever said this to us or even alluded to it, but it's how I felt. We have great friends through our kids' activities. Without policies and procedures within each organization it falls to parents of food allergic kiddos to be on top of this. Our normal is different from everyone else's.

One year I reached out to the Little League President in our town and tried to explain some of this. I asked if there might be an opportunity for me (little old me, local food allergy mom with no certification or anything beyond experience and drive) to address all the coaches at the start of the season. He said they'd be having a mandatory coach's meeting soon and I was welcome to speak for a few minutes. Yay! Perfect! Then he told me the date and time. Gah. I already had a commitment at that time and could not attend. COVID hit before the next season, derailing any of these plans.

In all honesty, though, the idea felt overwhelming. Was I really going to try to reach out to every sports program in the community and show up to educate their coaches about food allergies? I was overwhelmed thinking about it, which means nope, I probably wouldn't have. I didn't have the answer, but I believed that with a big picture change we could increase education and awareness, and ultimately, more uniform, safe inclusion throughout activities. I was still "just a food allergy mom," but it was always in the back of my mind. I believed in my heart there was a way. A way that meant moms who were not signing their kids up for programs,would feel comfortable doing so. Would trust that there was a best practices plan in place that considered food allergies (and any other disabilities).

I feel like I have to elaborate just a tad here. This idea of safe inclusion can be confusing. If a kid is safe and they are included, we're all good right? No, it's not that simple. Safe inclusion to me is when a child is included, to the greatest extent possible, the same way as their peers, and that their safety is non-negotiable. We have a free, local after-school program right now that I spend a lot of time thinking about in this regard. They provide snacks to all the kids and keep a stash of safe snacks so any child who attends always has a safe option. It's awesome! But sometimes they plan "special snacks" like pizza parties and ice cream sundaes. So while most kids are devouring ice cream sundaes and slices of pizza you have other kids noshing on fruit snacks or safe granola bars. Safe? Yes. Included? Well, this is where I will argue no. The "special snacks" are a highlight of the program. It is used to get kids in the door. I can appreciate wanting to increase participation, but because my passion lies in the safe inclusion of food allergic individuals, this increased participation comes at the cost of some kids. It fires me up when some people's needs are put ahead of others. In my honest opinion, if it excludes any child, then it is not best practice. Best practice meaning safe and equitable inclusion. If that's not possible, consider choosing something different. Safe and equitable inclusion might require communicating with families ahead of time. It might mean cross referencing a list of allergies and restrictions from the school nurse and avoiding anything on the list. It might even mean changing course and planning a special activity instead of a special food item. No matter what, it's possible. I've come across naysayers who wave their hands at this kind of thinking and say, "the world can't change for these kids, they have to learn to get over it and move on. They can't expect everyone to bend over backwards for them." Bear with me as I try to make a rough, but hopefully relatable, comparison. Imagine an event where everyone is given a brand new Apple Watch. Oh, but not you. You were born with oversized wrists and the Apple Watch won't fit yours. It's not your fault of course, you were born this way. So that you are not left out, they have a special rubber bracelet that will fit your wrist. It's well made, and it means you get to have something on your wrist just like everyone else. But, come on. Apple Watch versus rubber bracelet? Ice cream sundae versus a piece of fruit? Sure, you can argue that not all kids like Apple Watches or ice cream. First, that's not the point, and second, *at least they have the choice.* When you make a choice for someone else it's different. Is childhood not hard enough? Why would we make it harder for any child?

I think to truly determine if safe and equitable inclusion is happening we need a good definition of inclusion and equitable. Here's one.

> Merriam Webster – Inclusion: the act or practice of including and accommodating people who have historically been excluded (as because of their race, gender, sexuality, or ability).[40]

In this context, safe inclusion means changing how we approach food use so individuals are no longer excluded because of their food allergies. Historically it has been acceptable to give food allergic kids a safe but separate seat in the lunchroom, or a safe but different and usually less exciting food item so they "have something." We can do better. Through education and awareness I believe we can make safe inclusion the norm. Safe and not meant to feel different. Here's another one.

> Merriam Webster – Equitable: dealing fairly and equally with all concerned.[41]

---

40. Merriam-Webster https://www.merriam-webster.com/dictionary/inclusion
41. Merriam-Webster https://www.merriam-webster.com/dictionary/equitable

This will take a conscious commitment. Awareness and education are key for progress with this. I think a great way to work on this is by educating children. Let's teach them best practices and empower them to do better. When I was a classroom teacher one of my students was on the Autism spectrum. Early in the year, and with her son's permission, his mom scheduled a time to come in and speak to my class. She wanted to help his classmates understand him better. She didn't want them wondering, talking about him, making their own assumptions, or bullying him. She educated them briefly and age appropriately and then she invited them to ask questions which she kindly and patiently answered. Thanks to her effort, this group of students had increased compassion. She empowered them as peers.

> "Children are the world's most valuable resource and its best hope for the future." ~John F. Kennedy

I have seen how kids can rise to the occasion given the opportunity. How they can step up as allies for their peers. I'm not saying all kids all the time, but I am saying it's possible. After my school district adopted the new policy and procedures around life-threatening food allergies I was asked to help develop a curriculum for the elementary health program. I was happy to help. With the support and guidance of our district's Health and Wellness Chair, I spent a few months creating a program we called AWARE to be used in grades K-5 the following school year. I often see food allergy kids' friends become their allies, and empowering these friends with knowledge requires just a little teaching. Teach them some background, teach them how to be a helpful friend, and teach them what to do if something happens.

Teacher feedback of the AWARE program was mediocre. Out of all the lessons, there was one favorite by far. It was the one about hand washing and I got it – it was my favorite too. It was the most fun and, as we've covered, kids like to have fun! In the end, COVID and budget cuts prevented further use of the curriculum.

One day a flyer came home from the Recreation Department advertising two classes that would be offered during school vacation week. They were offering both a Staying Home Alone Class and a Babysitter Training Class. What a great idea! I wondered if they covered food allergies so I called them. I had a lovely conversation with one of the co-founders, Bette Antonellis. She invited me to join her and her business partner, Denise Laiosa, for coffee. I had a really nice time getting to know them. I learned more about their classes, and that they touched slightly on food allergies and epinephrine use. They were interested in what I could share about food allergies. I signed Shea up for the Staying Home Alone class a few weeks later and they invited me to attend and listen. I parked myself discreetly in the back of the room hoping not to distract the kids. When they reached the part where they were talking about allergic reactions and epinephrine auto-injectors, they invited me to come up and demonstrate for the class how to use an epinephrine auto-injector. I enjoyed the opportunity and was excited to continue the conversation with them. They were connecting with and educating kids and families in the community already. There was so much I could learn from them!

A consistent challenge for me over the years was "trying not to freak people out." Freaking out babysitters as I tried to calmly explain about my kids' food allergies, how to manage them, and what to do in case of emergency. Freaking out other parents as I tried to calmly explain and hand over the epinephrine auto-injectors before a playdate. I say "I tried to calmly explain" because inside I was not calm. I was nervous every time and I'm sure that came through. I always felt like there had to be a better way, I just didn't know what it was.

Then it hit me one day. What if there was a training program for babysitters to learn about food allergies? What if there was a specific time and space where they could learn, ask questions, and gain confidence around caring for kids with food allergies? What if parents like me didn't have to feel that nervousness around freaking others out? I shared my idea with Bette and Denise and they encouraged me to create a class that I could pilot under their business, South Shore Safety. What an awesome opportunity! I got right to work developing a Babysitter Food Allergy Training class. I focused on prevention and preparedness efforts, which Dr. Pistiner teaches as the two pillars of food allergy management. This would be that "better way" I had imagined all those years before. I believed variations of this class, and the information in it, could be useful for educating other groups as well. I felt like there was a lot of good work I could start doing. Bette and Denise started advertising my Babysitter Food Allergy Training class to communities they had worked with before, but sadly COVID hit and it all came to a screeching halt. This work was put on the back burner. I dusted it off every now and then and added different versions of classes to my collection, knowing there would be value to it when the time came

A consistent goal for me with each of these endeavors was to help food allergic children be more safely included. Meaning, those around them have been educated just enough to help make areas of life better than they would have been before. Things got easier as communication increased. After brainstorming with our church's Director of Religious Education, she invited me to do a lesson at the start of the church year for the kids. I reviewed the basics of the AWARE program. Time hasn't always allowed, and COVID put a pause on this for a couple years, but doing hands-on lessons would be more fun so I hope to incorporate that in the future.

I enjoy finding educational opportunities through my work with SAFE. Each year I am able to propose a project and apply for a COA from FARE. COVID got in the way, but I tried to find virtual options in 2020 and 2021. In 2022 I organized a week-long trivia contest which was fun and we had a great number of participants. Each day, those who answered correctly were entered into a random name picker to win a gift card. We also did a Halloween Costume Contest and everyone who provided a picture of their costume and told us what they do to stay food allergy safe on Halloween (for educational purposes) won a prize. We shared these ideas with our SAFE community in the hopes that some families might find new, useful, and/or helpful ideas from other families. I loved being able to provide prizes and loved celebrating things related to food allergies. These fun engagement activities allowed families and kids to focus on some of the positives around their food allergy management instead of the all too common focuses around fear, exclusion, and stress.

Additional ways to increase education in the community would be through improved legislation. I've advocated for multiple food allergy bills at the state level over the years, at times giving in-person testimony and other times submitting written testimony. I have been fortunate that my local legislators have been supportive each time I've contacted them about legislation. My Senator, Patrick O'Connor, has been terrific. He or someone from his team always responds when I reach out and he has supported all legislation I've contacted him about. I am grateful to know I can reach out when the food allergy community needs support. It's rewarding to help make an impact on the larger community. Legislation around Massachusetts restaurants has been an area of interest. My friend, Nicole Arpiarian, started working on restaurant legislation after her son had an anaphylactic reaction in a

Boston Restaurant. Her patience, persistence, and politeness have made her a great advocate. She's the first to say she had no idea what to do when she started out, but she saw a need and just kept going, one step at a time. There is attention around the cost of epinephrine auto-injectors. Some states are capping the price. I look forward to supporting proposed legislation here in Massachusetts. It's worth looking to see if your state has proposed legislation around this. If so, it will need your support. Get talking about it. Bring it to people's attention. Connect with your local legislators and ask for their support. Offer testimony when possible. You can support change.

Over the years I had become aware of more and more women in Massachusetts working in their communities around food allergies in one capacity or another. Lauren and I met with some of these women and soon realized there were even more. We decided to contact the women we knew of who were active in the food allergy space and try to get all of us together. This group included Kristie DeLoreto (a food allergy mom who started a non-profit on the North Shore to promote awareness around food allergies and asthma. Lauren and I attended one of her fundraising galas a few years ago which was inspiring), Erin Brazil (a Boston food allergy mom who has been active in the community and started one of the biggest Facebook groups in the area for food allergy parents, No-Nuts Moms Group, Boston), Emilé Baker (a food allergy mom who worked to improve the schools in her community and is also a therapist. Part of her practice is now focused on supporting parents managing food allergies, which is wonderful. She can be found in The Food Allergy Counselor Directory). Anna White (a dedicated and active food allergy mom in Boston), Nicole Arpiarian (our fearless advocate working on restaurant legislation), Nicole Hartery, Vicki Gifford, and Rania Hito were all food allergy moms trying to make a difference. Trying to make life better for their kids and beyond. A date was set and as many of us as was possible came together to meet and brainstorm in real life (most of us meeting for the first time) – what were the biggest issues we saw and how did we think we could partner to make positive change? It was amazing. I joked that this group was like Target's big red "Easy" button. One call and we could access each other quickly. We met a number of times, first in person and then via Zoom (before Zoom was a thing). We called ourselves the Food Allergy Leaders Association (FALA). Together we wrote a Mission Statement: "FALA strives to improve quality of life for the food allergy community by building a strong collective voice and empowering those touched by food allergies." Our biggest strength was our partnership. When COVID hit our work came to a screeching halt. While many of our ideas never came to fruition, we are still connected and able to hit that big red button if we need to. This powerhouse group of women is a gift. I am grateful knowing they are there to ask questions of, share ideas with, or ask for their support. And, I am ready to do the same for them.

Hitting the Road

"The greatest legacy we can leave our children is happy memories." ~Og Mandino

My comfort with travel as a food allergy mom fluctuated. Early on we traveled a decent amount, always by car. I would drive three hours to visit my parents without thinking twice. We would drive five hours to visit extended family. We would travel to Cape Cod for a week with Jay's family. I craved adventures.

When Shea ended up in the ER in New York on her first Thanksgiving I was terrified, but it felt like an isolated event. I didn't "get it" yet. As the kids got older I started to think to myself "this is hard." Each trip we took required more planning and preparation than in our previous life, and more than what was required of friends and family. Travel came to mean more work and more stress than just staying home. We lost the ability to be spontaneous and I was losing my excitement for travel because it felt daunting.

When out of town friends invited us to visit for the day, I'd look for excuses. They were excited to catch up and see our kids play together, but all I could think about was how food would impact the visit. Too many times I had been mentally exhausted during a visit because I was trying to act normal while in reality I had to stay completely tuned in to the kids. I would carefully and discreetly position myself between the kids if their kiddos were eating goldfish (or pizza, or mac-and-cheese, or peanut butter and jelly, or any number of "normal" kid foods). Then I'd have the awkward task of asking if they wouldn't mind washing their kids' hands after they ate so my kids wouldn't break out in hives. I knew it was important and I never had a friend who pushed back, but it still wasn't my favorite thing to do.

You worry you sound crazy. You worry you sound rude. You worry people are judging you and you also feel alone. I wasn't confident yet as a food allergy mama. I was still trying to be "normal." Well folks, if you haven't heard, there's no such thing as normal!

FIRST FLIGHT

In 2014 Dana and her family moved to North Carolina. I was sad to see them go. I traveled down to celebrate her birthday one year, and she came to visit with the kids at another point. Eventually we had an opportunity to visit them as a family and I really wanted to go – but I was scared. How would we fly on a plane? How would we feed the kids when we arrived?

I was honest with her. I told her how badly I wanted to come and how much fun I knew it would be. But also, I was struggling with how to fly safely and feed them while we were there. Jay and I believed we could do it with the right planning.

Her daughter Kambrie has a peanut allergy so they weren't new to food allergies. Dana had watched Shea years before when Thomas went to the hospital for his peanut butter reaction. She and I had done those cooking nights years ago, too, which allowed our kids to eat together. We talked about how we could make this work.

She agreed to take me to the store as soon as we arrived, that way I could focus on getting safe food without the kids around and she could help me. We came up with a meal plan for the stay so we knew what to buy. She was so helpful in making the trip a success, but it required me to be honest and vulnerable with her. I hadn't always felt comfortable doing this with others.

Before we left I did some research on flying with food allergies. There were no rules about the "right way" to do it. I read, learned, and picked things we could try. Like, letting the crew know our children had food allergies so we could board the plane early. This allowed us to wipe down the seats and trays before anyone else got on the plane. It seemed like a great idea at the time. The only problem was that our seats weren't very far back on the plane, and right after they let us on they let everyone else start boarding. It was a traffic disaster!

There we were wiping things down with our two little kids standing by watching. We were holding up traffic and getting the evil eye along with huffing and puffing from perfect strangers. It was humiliating, frustrating, and embarrassing. All we could do was wipe faster hoping we got all the nooks and crannies. I had also heard that you should make sure the plane announces your kids' allergies so everyone knows. Well, they did and truth be told, it was embarrassing. Our seats were such that we were in separate rows one behind the other. The kids each had a window seat and Jay and I each had a middle seat. The people sitting on the other side of us posed no risk. At no time did I feel like my kids would have been in danger, even if the other people were eating dairy or nuts.

After reflecting on these accommodations we decided that moving forward they weren't beneficial to our family. Based on the research we had done it seemed risky not to board early and not to have an announcement made. In hindsight I realized everyone has a different risk tolerance level and people make different decisions. We cleaned our area to prevent contact reactions. We packed safe snacks. We packed epi. We had learned from Dr. Pistiner that an allergen's protein would have to become aerosolized and inhaled if it were to impact my kids. If the crew was steaming milk in close proximity that could be an issue or if someone was making a whey protein shake in close proximity and the powder was in the air directly around my kids, that could be a problem. A sandwich or snack being eaten by another passenger didn't pose a risk to our kids. We used facts to combat some of our fears.

After this experience we started booking seats further back on the plane when possible, and boarding with everyone else. We didn't announce that our kids had allergies unless something came up where it would have made sense to. I had my kids wear long sleeves and pants to minimize skin contact with the seats, and we wiped things down once we sat. I kept wipes in an easily accessible location so we could pull them out and wipe arm rests, buckles, trays, screens, and anything else that made sense. It was more manageable, less embarrassing, and seemed to offer enough protection. I've met families who use a twin size fitted sheet and cover the seat from top to bottom. A big help for me has been hearing a variety of approaches over the years. Hearing from other families that there isn't a one size fits all approach made me feel better about making our own decisions. What works for my family might not be best for yours, but I hope it helps to hear some ideas.

SEDONA

When I was pregnant with Shea I had the unique opportunity to drive cross country with my sister Molly, including an unexpected few days in beautiful Sedona, Arizona. I called Jay each night from Sedona telling him what an amazing place it was, and how we just had to come back some time together. When the kids were little I told them stories about Sedona. I showed them pictures and shared what I loved about the natural beauty there. I would always say "I can't wait to take you there."

And yet the reality of those words overwhelmed me. How on earth could we take them there, safely?

In 2019 Jay and I decided it was time. We had saved up for it, and the rest came down to logistics. We were ready to make our Sedona dream a reality and decided to stay at the same place I had stayed all those years ago. It was a condo with a full kitchen so we could be independent with food. We researched local grocery stores and to our surprise there was a Whole Foods down the street, which was a familiar store with familiar brands. I will cover this later, but at this time in her life, Shea was experiencing some significant anxiety related to her food allergy and eating. At the time we didn't realize that by helping her avoid hard things, like unfamiliar foods from stores or restaurants, we were making things worse in the long run. But, for this trip, we tried to keep things easy for her. And for us.

We knew in advance there were some familiar foods we wouldn't be able to get there, so we looked into how to travel with food. Some people suggested ordering and shipping food ahead of time but I wasn't sure how that would work. Instead, we brought a carry-on cooler bag, packed tight with frozen foods our kids enjoyed. We figured it would stay cold and not spoil. It worked really well! We also packed a lot of non-perishable snacks in our suitcases. This also worked out great. Our grocery shopping in Sedona was primarily fresh fruits and veggies, but also meats, and refills of anything that made sense. It felt stressful ahead of time but once we came up with an organized plan and understood what was allowable with the airlines, we were confident.

We made sure we always had food, water, hand wipes, Benadryl, and epinephrine. Epinephrine has to be kept between 68 and 77 degrees Fahrenheit,[42] which is a serious challenge on hot summer and cold winter days. I knew Sedona would be hot and we would be outdoors quite a bit. Sticking their epi in a backpack would not suffice. We weren't bringing a cooler on hikes so I had to get creative. One thing we always brought was water and we carried a couple backpacks for water bottles. We decided to use two stainless steel, insulated water bottles to store the epi while we hiked. They worked great. The heat didn't get in. I've also heard Frio is a great product to keep epinephrine auto-injectors at safe temperatures.

> ### Frio
>
> The FRÍO® insulin cooler keeps in-use insulin and other temperature sensitive-medications cool and safe, within safe temperatures of 18-26°C (64.4-78.8°F) for a minimum of 45 hours, even in a constant environmental temperature of 37.8°C (100°F)
>
> frioinsulincoolingcase.com

We made memories of a lifetime and there was so much more to the week than food. Sure, some moments are tricky. During a day trip to the Grand Canyon we ran out of food for Shea. Her lunch "didn't taste right" (kids!) so she wouldn't eat it. She had become incredibly limited in what she was

42. Astham & Allergy Network "Epi storage tips at home and on the go" https://allergyasthmanetwork.org/news/epi-storage-tips-home-and-the/

willing to eat and was unwilling to eat any of the other food I had on hand. I was extremely frustrated with her. And scared. We were kind of in the middle of nowhere. We didn't trust going to a restaurant and we couldn't find a grocery store. We managed to get a banana at a gas station. I mean kind of eww, and random, but it worked. (I keep that day in the back of my mind, and since then I have tried to find non-perishable food items to keep in my purse or the glove compartment or her backpack. Some favorites include Chomps meat sticks and Enjoy Life protein bites.)

A special food related part of the trip came at the very end. A few months before our trip I had heard about a restaurant in Phoenix that was top eight free. Since we were flying in and out of Phoenix I made the plan for us to visit before we caught our flight home. It's called Intentional Foods, or IF. It's a restaurant and market. I was actually shaking as we walked in. We had never been anywhere like this and it seemed too good to be true. I introduced my family to the owners and told them we had come from Boston. I teared up when I was talking to them. They were so sweet and came out from behind the counter for hugs and pictures and a brief opportunity to connect. One of their children has food allergies and that's what prompted them to open IF. As they say on their website, "What IF everything on your favorite menu was allergy-friendly? What IF everything was both safe and delicious to eat? What IF friends and families could eat at one table?" Thomas was beside himself when he realized he

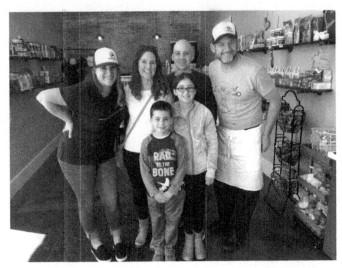

The Neri family in 2019 with Lisa and Ned Heath, owners of Intentional Foods (IF) in Mesa, Arizona

could literally order ANYTHING on the menu. He teared up. This had never in his life been an option. He was overwhelmed and wanted to order it all! Shea on the other hand struggled to wrap her head around it. She just couldn't believe it was safe. She chose not to get anything. It was too hard for her to believe that they really didn't have dairy in there somewhere. I think if we lived locally she would have come around to the idea. I felt badly since she had just this one chance, but I also knew that was her comfort level at the time. Thomas devoured his meal! We bought a few allergy friendly snacks from their market before thanking them and saying goodbye. Today, IF is free of the top nine allergens and they continue to shed light on allergy friendly brands in their market.

Overall our trip to Sedona was incredible! I'm proud we made it a priority even though we knew it came with challenges. If you are able, I encourage you to make a plan and hit the road with your family, to whatever place it is you want to visit. There are Facebook groups for traveling with food allergies, like the Allergy Travels Group. Usually, there is a way to make it happen safely. Learn from those who have gone ahead of you and pick up as many tips as you can to make things easier. The memories will be priceless.

WEDDINGS

My kids have been in more weddings than most! When Shea and Thomas were little we had four family weddings that we were part of and had to travel for. For my sister-in-law Pam's wedding, we communicated with the venue ahead of time so we knew the meal would be safe, which was great. I brought a backup meal just in case, but we didn't need it. Dessert was different. The cake wasn't going to be safe so we just brought safe cake slices from home and all went well. We had a stash of safe snacks that came in handy, too.

When my sister Maura got married on Cape Cod we stayed at my mom's beach house so we could have access to a full kitchen, which worked out well. We spoke with the caterer to determine which food items would be safe at the reception, and again brought extra food and safe desserts so Shea and Thomas had plenty to eat.

My sister Molly got married on Block Island, which, if you're not familiar with it, is a beautiful, quaint New England island off the coast of Rhode Island. It's lovely, but boy was I anxious about being on a small island in a hotel room without a kitchen. Gulp. We would be arriving by ferry with limited options once we were on island, so this trip required some serious advanced planning. We contacted the hotel and for a daily fee they put a small refrigerator in our room. It was smaller than the fridge I had in college but better than nothing. Every few hours or so either Jay or I trekked to the ice machine to replenish the ice in our cooler, which was acting as a second fridge. We brought a microwave which allowed us to heat the food.

Weeks prior, I had invested in partitioned food containers and spent the days leading up to the trip cooking and portioning out every single meal the kids would eat over the three day trip. We planned all their favorite meals so they would be excited rather than feel left out. While I am a big proponent of safe inclusion so kids are safe and feel like they belong, it's not always possible. That's a reality. In this case safe inclusion meant participation, it didn't mean eating the same food. They ate the food from home but it was important that we brought their favorites. It made the fact that their food was different a non-issue. We let them watch TV when they were eating in the room, something they weren't allowed to do at home. It felt important to make sure the experience was fun and special for them. At each meal we heated their food and quickly transported it to wherever we were gathered. The Rehearsal Dinner was at a restaurant down the street so we heated their food and trekked it down the hill. The wedding

To Include or Not to Include

To include or not to include, that is the question. In my family's experience, there are times when it makes sense to eat the same food as the people we are with, and there are times when it doesn't. Every situation is different and everyone's comfort level is different so we usually look at each scenario uniquely before making a decision. Doing something because we felt pressured to never usually worked well. Even if it worked out safely, my anxiety level didn't justify the potential risk. Respect yourself and listen to your gut. Make the best decision you can based on the information you have at hand, in the moment.

reception was in the hotel so it was easy to run back and forth to the room for their food. When the cake was served, we pulled out their safe cake from home. Jay took much of the brunt of this process because I was in the wedding party. We didn't take chances and everything they ate came from home. It wasn't easy, but it worked, and we enjoyed the wedding!

CAPE COD RENTAL

Before having children, Jay and I vacationed in the summer with each of our families. Beach people on both sides! It was great to be together and I looked forward to starting a family so we could share all of it with them. The reality was more challenging than I ever imagined. Sharing a kitchen with a group of people who don't manage nut and milk allergies on a daily basis is hard. I'm sure it wasn't easy for them either. It felt harder as the kids got older because we knew more and we worried more. When COVID hit we were unable to go away with either side of the family so the four of us went away. The number one requirement for where we would stay was to have a kitchen. It still took planning and preparation, like researching local grocery stores and bringing foods we didn't know if we would find.

We had learned about the potential for cross-contact from kitchen supplies. Risky spots like uncleaned refrigerators, microwaves, tables, counters, toasters, silverware, plates, pots, pans, and glasses. Shea didn't forget this. At the time she still had a lot of anxiety about using a foreign kitchen and all that came with it. So we wiped and cleaned and washed and gave her a space that she felt more comfortable in. At the time I think she had the habit of washing every plate and utensil before use. Though it was never brought up by any of the therapists she had seen, I wonder if she had developed some OCD due to her anxiety. She leaned on a number of maladaptive and ritualistic behaviors to help herself feel safe, though, at the time, I didn't understand what was going on.

There were things about a foreign kitchen we really did need to be careful with. Like pans and cutting boards with deep scratches, where food debris can get caught and pose a risk. So we didn't use anything that looked concerning and sometimes we used tin foil to create a safe layer for cooking. This is a trick that has worked well for us over the years. If we go to a cookout for instance, we bring tin foil. It keeps it separate physically and is a good visual reminder for whomever is manning the food. Often Jay jumps in to cook the kids' food.

We use separate plate and utensils for taking their food off the grill. In our case, it's cheeseburgers that tend to be the biggest threat on a shared grill. Good communication has worked well in those instances, and tin foil continues to be a helpful tool when we are cooking away from home.

This vacation was different from the family vacations of years prior. It was certainly easier not having to manage meals and a kitchen with others, but we missed the fun and magic that comes with staying in a house with extended family. The kids missed their cousins. The following year we found a balance by taking some time as just the four of us but then also joining the bigger family vacation again. Our precautions change depending on the type of trip. We have no choice but to plan and prepare. But then, it's important to enjoy the ride. Make the plans and, most importantly, make the memories.

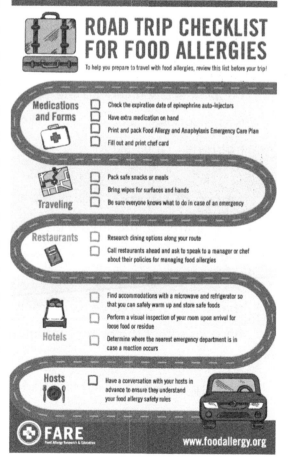

ROAD TRIP CHECKLIST FOR FOOD ALLERGIES

To help you prepare to travel with food allergies, review this list before your trip!

Medications and Forms
- Check the expiration date of epinephrine auto-injectors
- Have extra medication on hand
- Print and pack Food Allergy and Anaphylaxis Emergency Care Plan
- Fill out and print chef card

Traveling
- Pack safe snacks or meals
- Bring wipes for surfaces and hands
- Be sure everyone knows what to do in case of an emergency

Restaurants
- Research dining options along your route
- Call restaurants ahead and ask to speak to a manager or chef about their policies for managing food allergies

Hotels
- Find accommodations with a microwave and refrigerator so that you can safely warm up and store safe foods
- Perform a visual inspection of your room upon arrival for loose food or residue
- Determine where the nearest emergency department is in case a reaction occurs

Hosts
- Have a conversation with your hosts in advance to ensure they understand your food allergy safety rules

FARE
Food Allergy Research & Education

www.foodallergy.org

Well Hello There, Anxiety

"It takes courage to choose hope over fear."
~Mark Zuckerberg

Anxiety was coming at me from every direction. In the house, out of the house, my own and Shea's. Not having the foundational constant of one allergist played into this. Most people I know have had the same allergist since their child was diagnosed, but we were allergist hoppers transferring from one to the next for one reason or another.

A SEED PLANTED

After we moved to our new home, I wasn't impressed with the first allergist we saw at the satellite office, so I scheduled the kids' next annual visit with another doctor in that practice who came recommended by a neighbor. He was fine but within the next year I learned that Dr. Pistiner (who had led the workshop for parents at Children's Hospital years prior) had taken a job at Mass General Hospital for Children in Boston as the Director of Food Allergy Advocacy, Education, and Prevention in the Food Allergy Center. Additionally, he was taking new patients. I had been following Dr. Pistiner for years by this point, traveling to hear him speak whenever an opportunity presented itself. I'd been to hospitals and schools to hear him. I used to joke that I was a "groupie." As far as I was concerned, he was the best pediatric allergist in the greater Boston area. Upon hearing about his new position, I reached out to his office and initiated the transfer of my kids to his care ahead of their next annual allergist appointment.

After reviewing Thomas's test results he suggested an oral challenge with almonds. Yay! For years I had hoped we could try getting some of the nuts into his diet. After only a few years things were changing in the food allergy world. In the years to come I would begin hearing more and more about allergists encouraging food challenges, but when my kids were little it wasn't commonplace. It wasn't lost on me that years prior I was that crazy, borderline negligent mom who had threatened to feed her son nuts in the hospital parking lot, and now we were being invited into one of Boston's best hospitals to do the same thing. *Bring it on*, I thought. It would be awesome if he passed and we could introduce almonds into his diet. Some light in what had felt like a dark tunnel.

Ignorance is bliss when it comes to oral food challenges. I was blissfully ignorant going into that appointment. I had no idea what we were getting into even though I was very excited. We arrived early in the morning (no small feat considering morning commuter traffic into Boston). I was instructed to bring almond butter and epinephrine. That's all I had been told. The process was carefully orchestrated with a tiny dose given followed by a set amount of time for observation, then a larger dose given, followed by observation time, and so on. I was clueless about how long this would take. I think we were there for four hours. It was a struggle to keep Thomas, then seven, occupied the whole time in a small room. I hadn't brought anything to help pass the time. Fortunately, we survived the boredom and he passed! We were told to incorporate almonds into his diet which we did primarily with almond butter. Up until that point we had only used sunflower seed butter.

A few months later Dr. Pistiner encouraged another challenge at the hospital for Thomas, this time with pecans. I was grateful the numbers from his testing were low enough to try getting pecans into his diet. And this time I wasn't so ignorant! I knew what to expect. Guess who packed the iPad this time?! Same process as last time with increasing amounts of pecan. He passed again. We were told to incorporate pecans into his diet. I wasn't sure how to do that since we don't eat pecans often, but I didn't really worry about it. A few weeks later we were encouraged to do a cashew challenge with him, this time at home. I was a little stressed doing it at home, but he passed. We were told to incorporate cashews into his diet. Almonds had been easy. Pecans and cashews were harder and we definitely didn't incorporate them well or often. I later learned that if you don't maintain foods from previously passed challenges in the diet, the body can reject them. Unfortunately, in the months that followed he reacted to both pecans and cashews so we had to stop giving them to him. I was seriously bummed out that my lack of understanding prevented him from keeping these foods in his diet. He remains allergic to both of these nuts today. Fortunately, we kept almonds in his diet which he still eats safely.

Along with suggesting these food challenges Dr. Pistiner also suggested we stop using Benadryl as part of the kids' allergy action plans. From the very beginning of our food allergy journey we had been told to use Benadryl when the kids had a reaction. If it didn't work, give another dose. For each of my children's early reactions we had relied on Benadryl. Even with prescriptions for epinephrine, I still had the sense that Benadryl was first, and only if things got "really bad" (I didn't really even know what that meant in the beginning) would we use epi. This new guidance came as a shock after ALL the times we had given our kids Benadryl. All those times they had vomited in a restaurant, or in a parking lot, or at someone's

Benadryl

When my kids were little we always gave Benadryl (an antihistamine) at the first sign of an allergic reaction. We used it so many times over the years. Guidance around this has changed since our early days. Different allergists have different thoughts around using Benadryl, so speak with your medical professionals. The organization "Kids With Food Allergies" has some discussion around this from a contributing allergist.[43]

43. https://community. kidswithfoodallergies.org/blog/food-allergy-faqs-top-questions-about-anaphylaxis-and-epinephrine

house. The reactions had never seemed severe enough to use epi, and Benadryl had always been our quick, easy answer. I liked having Benadryl available to us. It felt less scary. But Dr. Pistiner explained there was concern it could mask symptoms of anaphylaxis, potentially delaying the administration of epinephrine that might be necessary to successfully combat an anaphylactic reaction. Ok, I thought. If this is what the expert says, then this is what we will do. I was all in.

Just because I was "all in" didn't mean everyone in my family was on the same page. I was clueless to the seed of anxiety that had been planted in Shea that day. Like me, she liked how easy Benadryl was and she liked having it as an option. After hearing this new guidance, she started thinking back on all the times she had needed it, and had the harsh realization that if those same situations were to happen again, they would require epinephrine. Epinephrine felt scary. I believe she started to freak out inside. Our family was about to face some serious obstacles.

My own anxiety was high but I wasn't tuned into it. I had no understanding of anxiety and absolutely did not recognize what I was experiencing as such. Looking back, the signs were loud and clear. When things got hard or scary I retracted. I pulled back. I did less of whatever seemed risky. There came a time when I didn't allow anyone to cook for my kids outside our home. This was especially hard on the grandparents. The world outside our kitchen felt scary. A kitchen with milk or nuts seemed like a minefield and I didn't know how to ensure there wouldn't be cross-contact. I felt like a computer: Too much risk. Shut it down. Abort.

With nobody else cooking for them it meant Jay and I had a lot more on our plate (haha, pun intended). I don't enjoy cooking so I narrowed down a collection of basic meals that were safe and fairly easy, and put them on rotation. I never cooked multiple meals in a night. The thought of that felt like torture. We all ate the same thing for dinner. As long as they ate their dinner we allowed dessert. I used to tell my kids "you don't have to love it, you just have to eat it." They usually ate what I cooked without much trouble and today, I'm happy to report, they're both good eaters.

It was subtle at first. An innocent, "No thanks, I don't like those anymore." Then, "No thanks, I don't want to try that." Then, "No thanks. I don't want to eat what so-and-so made. I'll just have the leftovers in the fridge." Everyday life was happening around us so we didn't notice. But once it became inconvenient I sure started noticing. We had always been a one meal family for dinners and suddenly needing back-up plans with alternate food options was not convenient. Shea had developed an indescribable amount of fear around food. I felt guilty about this fear, like it wasn't fair that my child should have to be afraid of food. I thought following her lead was the best way to support her. If she didn't feel comfortable eating something I didn't push it. We thought we were helping. Unbeknownst to us fear was growing at a rapid rate inside her. She was desperate to avoid having an allergic reaction.

Family Meals

Basic family meals often included stir fries with chicken and a variety of veggies, Mexican dishes usually with chicken, fish, or shrimp, bean burritos, vegetable soup, chili, roasted veggies, a variety of types of chicken, broiled fish, pasta and meat sauce, BBQ chicken. I learned that almost anything tastes good when its roasted with olive oil, salt, and pepper. I got in the habit of making my own taco seasoning, chili seasoning, and salad dressing. They were safe, but also pretty dang tasty if I do say so myself. I eventually realized that making big batches of the seasonings simplified things for a while because they stored easily in mason jars and I didn't have to make them as often. I was always looking for ways to simplify life in the kitchen. We used dinner leftovers as lunch A LOT. Breakfast was typically eggs, veggies, maybe oatmeal with fruit, and treats like pancakes and bacon on weekends when we had more time. It was a lot of real food. When we found packaged foods that we trusted it made life easier. That said, there was never a guarantee, so we still had to use caution.

It's easy to see now that we could have handled this differently. Generally speaking, Jay and I have not parented in a "follow the kids' lead" way but we had been following her lead with this, trying to be kind and understanding. We felt bad for her. She was becoming an expert at avoidance. Avoiding new foods, old foods, and anything made outside our home. Then she started worrying about pots, pans, plates, silverware, and glasses at other people's homes. It was becoming challenging to plan overnights anywhere without preparing and packing every bit of food and silverware from home. She had never been like this before.

Then it got even harder. She started reacting to food. Familiar foods. Safe foods. "My throat feels funny," she would say with a scared look in her eyes. I would gently talk her through it, monitoring her for additional symptoms. We hadn't needed epi, but it was always close by. We started taking foods off the list of what she would eat. "My throat feels funny." OK, remove this food. "My throat feels funny." Ok, remove that food. In a very short time it seemed she had developed new food allergies. The list of foods she ate was getting shorter by the day. We reached a point where she was only eating seven foods on rotation. It was scary and stressful and I was worried the number would decrease further.

My head was spinning. She was scared and I'll be honest, so was I. One of the moms I had met a family through SAFE had told me about how her son had developed multiple new food allergies when he hit puberty. That's all I could think of. At age 10 this seemed feasible. It helped knowing this was a possibility though it terrified me to think it might be a reality. We needed answers to what was going on. We had our trip to Arizona coming up and I was starting to panic about traveling with her.

Getting back into Boston for appointments wasn't easy, so as much as I loved having my kids in Dr. Pistiner's care, I switched, yet again, to a more local allergist. She was unique in that she also managed asthma. This was helpful because around the same time, both Shea and Thomas were having flare ups of wheezing and asthma, which they each had a history of. It had always been managed by our pediatrician, but someone told me about this local allergist who managed asthma as well. She was great and helped us get their asthma under control.

It had only been a month since the kids' annual visit but I needed help. I called the allergist and they fit Shea in the next day. The first thing they did was weigh her, as they always did. I was stunned to see that she had lost six pounds in that time. Six pounds! As a small fourth grader she didn't have six pounds to lose. I desperately wanted to get the allergist's attention without alerting Shea. I know I've said it before but specialist visits with kids can be hard. To my relief the doctor noticed the weight change on her own and caught my eye. The gravity of the situation was hitting me. We had to find out right away what she was allergic to! This was an issue and we needed answers. She listened to everything we shared and came up with a list of potential culprits to test for.

The test results shocked us all. Negative. Shea wasn't allergic to anything new. I believe it was the allergist who told us that these "reaction" symptoms could actually be symptoms of anxiety.

Anxiety? For real? I'd heard of it, of course, but I had no understanding. It felt like I needed to become an expert, quickly. There are three meals a day and we were literally struggling at every single meal. Additionally, she started refusing to eat without me nearby and it was breaking my heart. She was so scared every time she had to eat. I didn't know what to do.

I filled Jay in after work. We were navigating uncharted waters. We were relieved she didn't have new allergies, but it was confusing and we were challenged by what to do next. How to help our sweet girl. My mom and I are very close so I called her that evening. She was sympathetic to our situation and knew we needed help fast. She immediately connected me to her dear friend who is an Integrative Holistic Psychologist in Connecticut, Dr. DeAnn Ewart. DeAnn agreed to speak with me over the phone at 8 AM the next morning. Literally before

Tapping – EFT

Research shows that tapping calms the amygdala in the brain, regulates our nervous system, and reduces stress and anxiety. Tapping is a powerful holistic technique based on the combined principles of ancient Chinese acupressure and modern psychology.[44]

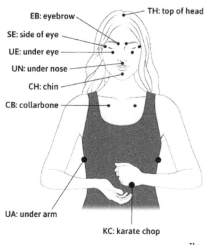

Tapping Points

EB: eyebrow
SE: side of eye
UE: under eye
UN: under nose
CH: chin
CB: collarbone
TH: top of head
UA: under arm
KC: karate chop

The Tapping Solution

44. Find more information at www.thetappingsolution.com

breakfast, which was the next meal. She understood that every mealtime mattered for us.

I am forever grateful to DeAnn for speaking with me that morning. Her patience, knowledge, and gentle approach helped me off a cliff. I was a terrified mom who had no idea how to help her child. She gave me a crash course on the brain and the mind. She helped me think about them in new ways and see some of what was happening instinctively with Shea, and what I could start helping her to reprogram. She stepped into our crisis during that call and gave me tools that gave us a fighting chance. She suggested using "Tapping," or Emotional Freedom Technique (EFT), to shift the neural pathways in Shea's brain. As soon as we hung up I got to work.

Things changed immediately, a tiny bit. I was blown away by the power the mind can have on the body. Literally, in time for breakfast I was able to talk and tap Shea through so she could stay calm and not "react." It required me to sit with her while she ate. She was scared to eat alone but fortunately she was open to the support.

This all happened shortly before our trip to Sedona, Arizona. I was more worried than ever about how to travel with her, but with DeAnn's help I felt like we could do it.

Everything was leading to fatigue for me. I was emotionally and mentally drained. Jay was incredibly supportive, but I was in the driver's seat and Shea was looking to me for strength every day. I needed to be in the right space to help her and I was struggling to bear the weight of it all.

Self Care for the Caregiver

Like with managing anything challenging, stress can take a toll. When my kids were little I had a membership to the gym. This was a game changer for me for a number of reasons. It was between meals so I didn't have to worry about food. We were in the same building so I felt much more comfortable than leaving them with a babysitter. I was taking time for myself. This mattered more than I knew. I got a break. I had a chance during the day to be "me," not just their "mom." I was using my body, working on my physical strength and endurance. I was prioritizing my health. I was also guaranteeing a shower! For anyone who has been a stay-at-home mom before, it is hard to get a minute to yourself. Later in my journey when we couldn't afford a gym membership, and again when COVID hit, I turned to power walking. My kids were older and either at school or Jay was home so it was easier to get out, but the movement, fresh air, and my competitive nature of trying to power walk a mile faster than the day before, got me out of my environment and was a form of self care. I know people who turn to massage, yoga, barre, dancing, and meditation just to name a few. The key is that it gets you out of the physical and/or mental space you spend most of your time, and you enjoy it. Like on an airplane, put your oxygen on first before you try to help others.

I needed help with her so I decided to find her a therapist. Much easier said than done. It was extremely challenging to find a practitioner who worked with kids, was taking new clients, *and* understood food allergies.

Years prior I had taken Shea into Boston for an appointment with Jennifer Lebovidge, who had led the workshop with Dr. Pistiner at Children's Hospital that we found so helpful. She is a wonderful person, and a dedicated professional. Unfortunately, the logistics of getting into Boston for regular appointments was just too difficult and we couldn't continue. So I contacted our pediatrician's office and asked for help. They put me in touch with a free local referral service that connected us with a more local therapist. She was young, which I thought would be great as she might be more relatable to Shea. Unfortunately it didn't last long. She was completely clueless to the intricacies of food allergy management. After she told Shea she had to, "go out to eat more often to get over your fear," I was like, ok, we're done here. Thanks so much for the help.

We started the search again. We were matched with a lovely woman. She bonded with Shea, who enjoyed going. They played games and talked about all sorts of things from what I could gather, but it wasn't "helping." I didn't have years to fix this, I needed help now. Shea was still afraid to try new foods and eat outside the house. I felt terribly alone and desperate for a team of helpers. Without a team I felt like I had to fix it. *But I'm not qualified*, I would think to myself. *I have no idea what to do*. I wanted to shout "Help! Help! SOS! Please, someone!" But no one came who could help. We were loved by so many, we knew that. Family, friends, but love wasn't enough. I needed someone who had experience with food allergies and this anxiety that didn't seem like any other anxiety I was aware of. This wasn't the fear of a plane crashing which is super highly unlikely, this was a fear of reacting to food when she had to eat multiple times a day. We needed someone who understood or at least respected the intricacies of this kind of anxiety and understood the sense of urgency we were facing.

My sister Maura is a family and child therapist. We talked about this multiple times. I would ask her why therapists aren't trained in certain niches. I figured food allergies aren't the only space where a need isn't necessarily being met. She didn't know. I shared that I would love to have food allergy trained therapists. Like, what if college students were alerted to areas of need, like this, so they could choose a focus for their studies? I knew that even if a program was developed tomorrow, it wouldn't be a quick fix but it certainly wouldn't hurt.

Our search for a therapist continued. I reached out to a fellow food allergy mom from SAFE who had confided in me that her teenage daughter was working with a therapist. Someone familiar with food allergies? Yes, please! I called the therapist and she apologized letting me know she was no longer taking child clients. What a bummer, I thought. But then she said something that stopped me in my tracks. "It must be hard to be the parent of a child with food allergies." I didn't know this woman but I suddenly felt seen. "Yes. Yes it is." I responded. "I am taking on new adult clients if you're interested." The rest is history. I have been working with Charisma ever since. She is not an allergy informed clinician in Tamara's Directory but she has helped me process a lot

The Food Allergy Counselor

I was thrilled when I first came across the Food Allergy Counselor Directory and Resources, started by Tamara Hubbard. This is exactly what I had been talking about and hoping for! Tamara is a therapist and a food allergy parent. She "gets it." She refers to those in her Directory as "Allergy Informed Clinicians."

Some data specific to quality of life (QoL):

- 92% of parents say they're always or occasionally fearful of their food allergic child's safety
- 75% of allergy parents reported that food allergies cause fear/anxiety for their family
- 1 in 4 parents report that food allergies causes a strain on their marriage
- Mothers rated their own psychological and physical QoL worse than fathers rated theirs; had higher scores than fathers for anxiety and stress
- Greater maternal overprotection was associated with lower child QoL as well as greater dietary and social limitations independent of food allergy outcomes
- 40% of parents reported experiencing hostility from other parents when trying to accommodate their child's food allergy

Given the common QoL impacts and increased anxiety experienced by those managing food allergies and allergic diseases, it makes sense that therapy services are a beneficial source of support. And just as therapists well-versed in other chronic and life-impacting health diagnoses such as diabetes and cancer, the allergy community benefits most from therapists who are well-versed in the basics of allergic diseases and the psychosocial/QoL impacts on lives. This data is a clear indication for a need for behavioral healthcare professionals to address this gap in psychosocial support for food allergy families. Tamara's Food Allergy Counselor Directory is an incredible resource. It is organized by state. With more and more therapists offering telehealth these days, hopefully it's becoming easier to find the support needed.[45]

45. The Food Allergy Counselor | https://www.foodallergycounselor.com/directory.html

over the years. She has helped me discover my own anxiety. Looking back, I'm sure that has impacted things along the way. More recently, and towards the end of writing this book, I learned I have ADHD which I'm sure has also impacted how I have mothered, how I have managed my children's food allergies, how I have managed it all. I am a work in progress. Aren't we all?

As I continued through the list of clinicians given to me I eventually found a local female therapist who worked with children. She, like my own therapist, was not an allergy informed clinician, but she said she understood anxiety and would do her best to help. Shea needed help beyond what Jay and I could give her and I was grateful to have another member on our team. This therapist supported our goal of getting new foods into Shea's diet, but months went by without much improvement. Whatever they were covering in sessions (I wasn't present) wasn't translating into everyday life. We managed to add a few foods but still had a long way to go.

You know how there are dates you'll never forget? Memories and moments forever ingrained in your mind. For my mom, it was the assassination of JFK. For me it had been Princess Diana's death and later September 11. You remember where you were and what you were doing, like it was yesterday. I've added March 13, 2020, to my list. Friday the 13th. The day our world "shut down." Schools closed for a long weekend, or so we thought. The COVID-19 pandemic had hit, and life got real weird, real fast. Schools stayed closed and the chaos of the unknown began. I was attempting to make masks at home thanks to YouTube videos, handkerchiefs, and hair elastics. Gloves were hard to come by. Waiting in line for an hour or more outside the grocery store, even in the rain, was suddenly a thing.

During COVID, Shea and her therapist transitioned to virtual sessions. Shea started asking if she could stop the sessions. We gave it some time, but eventually, and because we really weren't seeing a benefit, we stopped. We threw in the towel on therapy. It had been just about a year since the drastic and sudden weight loss and allergist visit that opened our eyes to the anxiety we were still very much navigating. A year. I knew we weren't at the finish line but I had no idea what to do next. And, COVID.

There was so much fear. So many new fears. Can I get food for my family? Will this invisible virus penetrate our home and hurt, or worse, kill, anyone in my family? Will we ever see our extended family again? Will we ever see our friends again? How do we stay safe? And really, nobody had answers for quite a while. We worked our way through those difficult days. Eventually we stopped washing our groceries before bringing them in and leaving mail in the garage for a few days for germs to "die off." The food allergy issues had taken a back seat.

Eventually we reached a new normal. For my family it was a calm we had not experienced previously. We reveled in the fact that we had less to worry about regarding food.

We had the safety and ease of a full time bubble – no lunch or snack time at school, no birthday parties, no family parties or holiday gatherings, no restaurants, no other kids with messy food. We settled in and appreciated the simplicity that pandemic life brought us.

But I think we can all agree, too much of a good thing isn't a good thing. Moderation is key. Avoiding food related challenges was nice and easy and all, but ultimately we were delaying our ability to be ready for the inevitable reopening of the world. We totally fell out of practice. For more than two years my family went to no restaurants, had no indoor family events, and no sleepovers with family or friends. Shea loved it. Her safe little bubble was there all day every day and we weren't asking her to do anything that made her uncomfortable.

When we went away that summer we made sure we stayed somewhere with a kitchen. We went to grocery stores and brought a lot of pre-made food. I tried suggesting new things. New food brands, new stores, new snacks, but she shot down anything that was new or different from what she was comfortable with. In my attempt to keep her safe, happy, and comfortable, I had inadvertently made things worse. In hindsight I could see this had been the wrong approach with her because our journey out of the COVID bubble was going to be much more difficult.

At some point I realized that if I didn't push Shea out of her comfort zone, nothing was going to change. She wasn't going to try new things on her own. Like a mama bird pushing her baby out of the nest, it had to happen. I had to help her move along. I was nervous because this wasn't what I was accustomed to as her mom. I knew she would push back fiercely due to her fears, which had strengthened over time. I had a chat with myself and committed to pushing her to try new, safe things – no matter what. I had to fake my own confidence to help her build confidence. This was really hard for me as a parent. I had been overprotective for years. I genuinely believed my choices along the way had been for good reason, but I was beginning to see I had prevented my child from learning to spread her wings. And so it began. Operation "Do the Thing" was *on*.

Her hesitation of new things was not limited to food. It was almost anything. Any suggestion I made or idea I had was met with "no" or the more creative "no way, not happening" and sometimes the "you can't make me!" Jay and I talked a lot in private, weighing the benefits of the things we were choosing to push on her. One such thing was a sexuality education class at our church for kids her age. For years I had heard wonderful things about this program and looked forward to when my children would be old enough to participate. We were still in the midst of COVID but a mini-version of the program was being offered. Teachers were in place and the plan was for the class to meet in person each week with masks on. My kids were still doing remote learning for school, so an in-person program brought up some feelings of discomfort, but we believed it was a safe approach and a great opportunity.

Of course she was like "no way!" and if I'm being honest EVERYTHING about this idea was hard for her. Jay and I were on the same page. This was safe, it was important, and it would be good for her. We just hoped it would be a positive experience so she wouldn't throw it back in our faces at the end! She wasn't alone. We were uncomfortable too, pushing her (forcing, she might say) into new things.

It was great! She may have been uncomfortable at times, but overall she got so much out of the experience and was very positive when talking about it. She felt safe and she enjoyed being in person with kids her age after so long. Upon the conclusion of the program, our Director of Religious Education, Tracey Newman, decided to host a celebration. Gulp. We had gone so long since dealing with food in social settings and now here it was again. Tracey emailed families with the suggestion of a pizza party and snacks to celebrate the end of the program. I replied and asked if we could find safe options since pizza wouldn't work for my kids. I will admit, I wasn't usually so bold asking for something different. Pizza is cheap and easy, I knew that. But I also knew this wasn't a large group and it might not hurt to ask.

She responded with, "No problem. Meghan, if you were organizing a gathering for your family where would you get food from?" I gave her the name of the local Chinese food restaurant we frequented. She said "Great, then we'll order from there. Give me a list of foods that are safe and that your kids like and I'll take care of it." Really?! I was overwhelmed by the kindness of this gesture. The celebration was so lovely, and my kids were able to eat almost all of what was available (there were additional items). Shea and Thomas made their plates first so there wouldn't be concerns with cross-contact. I was so grateful to Tracey and thanked her multiple times during the event. Eventually she said, "No need to thank me. This is what safe inclusion looks like." I was struck by this statement. She had been so supportive without making it feel weird. A lot of times, as hard as we try, food situations can get weird. It had been a long time coming, but she had a success under her belt!

Not long after the class ended, we rolled into summer. Jay found a day camp he thought the kids would enjoy. Fishing, hiking, kayaking, all the outdoorsy things. No food was involved which made it easy for us. It was every afternoon for a week. I wasn't sure this would be Shea's style, but Thomas was super excited so we pushed her to do it too. She was not interested, but fly little birdie, fly. We pushed her to go and she loved it! It was so good for her to push past her fear and anxiety leading to another success. These successes helped me too – I was becoming more confident with pushing her to do things she was reluctant to do.

Later that summer we signed Shea up for a week of drama day camp. She liked the idea but didn't want to do it. She was a nervous wreck. Thomas was too young so she'd have to go into this one alone. For years they had attended camp programs together. I understood her stress and anxiety.

This was new, this was uncomfortable, but we were on a mission to find things that COULD be done successfully. Camp had limited hours and didn't involve food. It was a topic she was interested in. It was close to home. She needed social interaction with kids who had similar interests. In my opinion it was perfect, but I had to push her hard to go that first day. And yes, you probably guessed correctly. She loved it. Things had been hard for her for so long and her anxiety had bled from food fears to basically anything different or new, even when food wasn't involved. It was a slow process and it wasn't easy, but she now had a third success under her belt. I cannot tell you how valuable that was as we rolled into the next school year. We used her successes as references each time something new and difficult came up.

When the next school year started there were new opportunities for her. "Why don't you join the yearbook committee?" I asked. "Ok." (Wow, that was easy.) "Why don't you check out School Council?" I asked. "Ok." "Why don't you do drama, they'll be putting on a play?" I asked. Well, even after multiple attempts I couldn't get her to agree to this one, but she had been trying so many new things in recent months that I let it go. Interestingly enough, when we went to see the play a few months later, she turned to me and said, "I really should have done drama." I just smiled. Next time.

In the spring of that year we learned the High School would be launching a girls golf team and they were opening it up to eighth graders to help build the program. She didn't know the first thing about golf but she said yes. And she loved it! The Universe kept rewarding her for being brave.

We eventually found another therapist who Shea worked with for a while. They had a great relationship and there was nothing wrong, but still it wasn't helping. We started having Shea work with an EMDR (Eye movement desensitization and reprocessing) therapist as well because I had heard it has even greater success with anxiety, but we saw no improvement. The only thing that was working was pushing her, supporting her, and celebrating her wins. And I'll be honest, giving her a phone. She felt significantly better when she knew she could call us when she was out in the world. It was an added layer of reassurance. She still doesn't say yes to everything, but it's been almost a year and she can talk about all the things she likes doing. She continues to blossom. She has so many more successes under her belt now, I could cry. Part of it is age and maturity, but much of it is finally DOING things. Where there's a will there's a way. This required us to commit to finding ways to do things safely so her world could expand. We considered, realistically, what the risks were (if any) and how we could prevent them.

We also learned to take some of her fears and talk to them. Call them what they were, and give them permission to leave her alone. Tell them they were no longer needed as part of her safety plan. At one point we were introduced to the workbook "What To Do When You Worry Too Much" and later "The Bouncing Worry Ball and Mighty Mitt." Both of which are good resources. We revisited tapping (EFT – refer back to page 205). There is a lot of information out there about this, but in simple terms you acknowledge that which is limiting you, give it permission to exist, and tell yourself you're ok anyway. It's freeing and encouraging and can open doors that have felt locked. Six months of regular tapping has shifted her from a tendency towards seeing only the negative to a stronger ability to see the positive. She is saying yes to things she never would have before. She is experiencing pride in ways she never before has. She has an easier time navigating difficult situations. It's been a great tool for her Life Toolbox.

In talking with other food allergy families and reading so many posts on social media, I noticed a theme of anxiety in far more families than just my own. One morning, about to head out for my daily walk, I decided to look up food allergy related podcasts. I happened upon an episode of The Itch Podcast about Managing Food allergy Anxiety. Their Guest Speaker was Lisa Rosenberg, M.Ed., MSW, LCSW, CSSW, who is a Food Allergy Counselor, Consultant, Educator, and Advocate. Lisa is a therapist who founded Safe & Included LLC, a food allergy counseling and consulting business. Lisa can be found in the Food Allergy Counselor Directory. I was so impressed by all Lisa had to say on the episode that I looked her up. And then I reached out to her. I wanted to connect with people like her and so many others who were doing incredible work within the food allergy space. As we chatted we came up with the idea that she could lead workshops for our Support

Group, which led to one of our biggest COA projects for SAFE. In the fall of 2021, Lisa led a series of three virtual workshops for SAFE – Food Allergy Anxiety, Food Allergies at School, and Food Allergies and Family Relationships. It was great and the sessions were well attended, which only reinforced the need for support around the mental health aspect of living with and managing food allergies.

The pandemic exposed how limiting fear and anxiety had made my family. It exposed our need to address the conflict between Shea's desire to live in a bubble forever, and a world of fun, interesting, exciting, unique, and wonderful things that were impossible to enjoy from inside a bubble. It probably would have been easier to address this when she was younger, but I hadn't seen what was happening. I hadn't understood. We'd had no modeling. I can see now that I had to address many of my own anxieties before I was able to help Shea with hers. It's never too late to make progress. We continue to work on this. Anxiety can feel debilitating, but I have hope that things can get better. My family focused on small steps, including tapping and saying yes to new things, but we also listened to and learned from professionals in the field. All of this helped us move in a healthier direction and begin to lessen the power anxiety had over us for so long.

Here We Go Again

"You are braver than you believe, stronger than you seem, and smarter than you think." ~A.A. Milne

Just one bite. That's all it takes. We know this. And yet it can happen so easily.

Nearly six years after Shea's anaphylactic reaction at my dad's wedding, it happened again. We spent a beautiful day on the beach with my sister Maura and her family. We had brought dinner, with plans to eat on the beach, but as can happen with Mother Nature, the winds shifted and it got cool. We decided to leave the beach and head to our house to enjoy dinner together there. The kids were excited to play but we first wrangled them to sit and eat. Then they could play and the adults could sit and eat.

Shea came over to me and said, "My throat feels funny." Ugh. Those words always give me a pit in my stomach. I tried to ignore it and stay light and positive to keep her from getting scared. So I simply said, "Aww, I'm sorry to hear that honey. Let's give it a few minutes and if you feel worse I can get you some Zyrtec. But, it might pass so let's see." (Our most recent allergist was on board with using antihistamines and suggested this over Benadryl to help minimize the drowsiness. For Shea, it helped lessen her anxiety. The allergist told us you can not mask anaphylaxis with antihistamine. It would never be strong enough, so we brought it back as an option.) She agreed but stayed right by me. Internally I was wracking my brain, was there something here that potentially caused a reaction? Everything we had made for dinner was familiar food she had eaten many times before and there was nothing of concern in my sister's kids' food. Deep breath, she probably just has a funny feeling that doesn't mean anything. Another deep breath.

After a few minutes she said, "Mom, I don't feel good," her voice wavering a little. She was nervous. She looked flushed. So I calmly said, "Ok, I'm going to go upstairs and get the Zyrtec. You're going to be just fine." Jay, Maura, and my brother-in-law Ryan were clued in to what was going on but none of us knew what was actually going on. They kept the other kids distracted and everyone kept their tones calm and light. She wouldn't leave my side so she came inside with me. Upstairs she started to cry saying she really didn't feel ok. I poured the little cup of Zyrtec for her and she downed it. I suggested we go back downstairs while we waited to see how she felt once it kicked in. We started down the stairs just as Jay was coming up. He let her pass and then he very quietly whispered in my ear, "there was milk in it." I looked at him with eyes wide open. I had to keep calm and not react the way I wanted to. I just stared at him and he said, "the fish sticks had milk in them."

We have been buying these fish sticks for years! Was it possible they suddenly had milk in them AND we missed it? We calmly continued down the stairs and while he stood at the kitchen island with Shea, I casually walked to our recycling bin to check the empty package. I thought I was cool, calm, and collected but she was watching me like a hawk.

"Why are you doing that? Why are you doing that?! Is there milk in them?! Is there!!??" It all happened at the same time. I saw the word milk listed in the ingredients, I became incredibly confused about how that could be, and Shea started to panic. To freak out.

Jay calmly went outside to tell Maura and Ryan so they understood and could keep the other kids outside, while I gently said to her, "Isn't that strange. Yes, milk is listed in the ingredients. I'm confused about how that happened but for now let's focus on you. I'm sorry you're not feeling well but I'm glad we know why. We know what you ingested and why you're feeling sick."

She was crying and still flushed. I said "I think we need to use your epinephrine." To which she responded, "No I don't want to." Moments like these are SO hard as a parent, but our years on this journey had prepared us for this. I knew better than I had at my dad's wedding. I had been educating myself for the last six years for exactly this type of situation. We were ready, even if we didn't want to be.

✚ FARE   FOOD ALLERGY & ANAPHYLAXIS EMERGENCY CARE PLAN

Food Allergy Research & Education

Name: _____ D.O.B.: _____

Allergic to: _____

Weight: _____ lbs. Asthma: ☐ **Yes (higher risk for a severe reaction)** ☐ No

PLACE
PICTURE
HERE

NOTE: Do not depend on antihistamines or inhalers (bronchodilators) to treat a severe reaction. USE EPINEPHRINE.

Extremely reactive to the following allergens:_____

THEREFORE:

☐ If checked, give epinephrine immediately if the allergen was LIKELY eaten, for ANY symptoms.
☐ If checked, give epinephrine immediately if the allergen was DEFINITELY eaten, even if no symptoms are apparent.

FOR **ANY** OF THE FOLLOWING:
SEVERE SYMPTOMS

LUNG
Shortness of breath, wheezing, repetitive cough

HEART
Pale or bluish skin, faintness, weak pulse, dizziness

THROAT
Tight or hoarse throat, trouble breathing or swallowing

MOUTH
Significant swelling of the tongue or lips

SKIN
Many hives over body, widespread redness

GUT
Repetitive vomiting, severe diarrhea

OTHER
Feeling something bad is about to happen, anxiety, confusion

OR A COMBINATION
of symptoms from different body areas.

1. **INJECT EPINEPHRINE IMMEDIATELY.**
2. **Call 911.** Tell emergency dispatcher the person is having anaphylaxis and may need epinephrine when emergency responders arrive.
- Consider giving additional medications following epinephrine:
  » Antihistamine
  » Inhaler (bronchodilator) if wheezing
- Lay the person flat, raise legs and keep warm. If breathing is difficult or they are vomiting, let them sit up or lie on their side.
- If symptoms do not improve, or symptoms return, more doses of epinephrine can be given about 5 minutes or more after the last dose.
- Alert emergency contacts.
- Transport patient to ER, even if symptoms resolve. Patient should remain in ER for at least 4 hours because symptoms may return.

MILD SYMPTOMS

NOSE
Itchy or runny nose, sneezing

MOUTH
Itchy mouth

SKIN
A few hives, mild itch

GUT
Mild nausea or discomfort

FOR MILD SYMPTOMS FROM MORE THAN ONE SYSTEM AREA, GIVE EPINEPHRINE.

FOR **MILD SYMPTOMS** FROM A SINGLE SYSTEM AREA, FOLLOW THE DIRECTIONS BELOW:

1. Antihistamines may be given, if ordered by a healthcare provider.
2. Stay with the person; alert emergency contacts.
3. Watch closely for changes. If symptoms worsen, give epinephrine.

MEDICATIONS/DOSES

Epinephrine Brand or Generic: _____

Epinephrine Dose: ☐ 0.1 mg IM ☐ 0.15 mg IM ☐ 0.3 mg IM

Antihistamine Brand or Generic: _____

Antihistamine Dose: _____

Other (e.g., inhaler-bronchodilator if wheezing): _____

_____

PATIENT OR PARENT/GUARDIAN AUTHORIZATION SIGNATURE   DATE   PHYSICIAN/HCP AUTHORIZATION SIGNATURE   DATE

FORM PROVIDED COURTESY OF FOOD ALLERGY RESEARCH & EDUCATION (FARE) (FOODALLERGY.ORG) 5/2020

Here's what I knew:

1. She had consumed her allergen.
2. She didn't feel well and had at least
    two symptoms at play.
3. Epinephrine would help her feel better.

All of this to mean: epinephrine was needed. As Lauren had said previously, it's like a house fire. Let's not allow it to spread by waiting to put it out. So I very confidently said, "We are going to do this and you'll be fine, I know you will." I went to the closet to get her Auvi-Q. What's unique about this brand of epinephrine auto-injector is that it talks to you. It is automated. Since we started getting this particular brand a few years ago, I've been reassured by this feature. For myself yes, but more so for others who may potentially need to help our children. It talks you through the process, how fantastic!

Well, reality was a different story. Stressful situations with a child aren't quiet and calm the way it had been any time we had practiced with the trainers. Shea was scared. She was crying and talking to us and we were talking to her and I couldn't hear a damn thing! Fortunately, I had practiced so many times over the years that it was fine. I knew what to do. I was confident. She was seated in a chair and I used the auto-injector on her outer thigh. We rubbed the area and hugged her and told her she was so brave and let her cry a little. Her response was great, "Wow, that didn't hurt nearly as much as I thought it would!" Phew, that made me feel better too. I said to her, "Ok I'm going to go call 911. They will probably want to take you to the ER to monitor you for a few hours so let's get you changed out of your bathing suit." Jay went upstairs with her to be close by so she wouldn't be alone. In hindsight this was not the best plan of action. We should have had her lay down until EMTs arrived. Fortunately she was ok.

I called 911. I surprised myself with how calm and level headed I was. I've called 911 more times in my parenting journey than I would have liked but all these years of learning had given me a foundation of knowledge and confidence for a moment like this. I knew exactly what to do. They said a crew would be right over and asked if I'd like them to stay on the phone with me. I was able to jokingly say that she was stable and with my husband so if it was ok I'd love to hang up so I could change out of my bathing suit and put on some real clothes!

The crew arrived within a matter of minutes, before Shea was back downstairs, in fact. Epinephrine after an allergic reaction is a funny thing. It works fast. She was feeling better already. When they came to the door I had to stifle a nervous laugh. "She's upstairs getting changed, she'll be right down."

As we had expected, they said they'd like to bring her to the ER for monitoring. The recommendation is to be monitored by medical professionals for about four hours because of the potential for a biphasic reaction. We agreed, and off we went in the ambulance. I was glad there were enough adults at my house to help Thomas and my nieces process what had happened, to keep them from being scared and worried about Shea. And, it certainly helped that Maura is a family and child therapist. I knew they were in good hands.

The hospital took her right back and she was hooked up to monitors. She had responded well to the epinephrine so far which was good. The nurse confided in me that she had a toddler with food allergies and this sort of thing scared her so much, even as a nurse. I told her about SAFE and gave her a business card. She joined our Facebook group that night. Her story was like so many I had heard before. Diagnosis, prescription for epi, and instructions to avoid. It's hard to "re-enter" the world after that. I knew she could find others to relate to in the group. If nothing else it's important to know you're not alone. You're not crazy when you feel like it's hard.

As the epi began to wear off symptoms started to develop again. Shea looked like she had a bad sunburn on her whole body, and it was itchy. I had heard of this sunburn type rash from food allergy mom friends but I had never seen it firsthand. She was also shaking uncontrollably and had been vomiting. I had to explain to her that the medicine helped right away but as it wears off her body is still

Biphasic Reactions

A variant of the usual monophasic (single phase) anaphylaxis, biphasic anaphylaxis is a well recognized presentation of the anaphylaxis syndrome. It consists of a recurrence of symptoms after an asymptomatic window in which patients seem to successfully recover from the first reaction. The second onset of anaphylaxis occurs without subsequent allergen exposure.[46]

46. "Biphasic Anaphylaxis: What You Should Know" - AllergyHome.org

processing the allergen. The ER doctor was great and willing to speak openly with me. It was clear she knew her stuff and I appreciated that she realized I knew my stuff too. We talked about options. While another epi injection wasn't to be ruled out, she was concerned about the shaking. I agreed. She decided to use a few other meds first to see how she responded. Fortunately it was a positive response and after a few more hours she was released. The doctor trusted that I knew what to watch for if the reaction resurfaced and that we would come back if need be. After a five hour visit we went home and got Shea comfortably into her own bed.

What?! How did this happen? Where had we failed? As Jay and I pieced it all together it became very clear what happened. All those years ago, Dr. Pistiner and Dr. Lebovidge had taught us that bringing safe food into your home is a three-step process. By making these three steps part of your routine you can most successfully manage a food allergy.

1. Check in the store that it's safe.
2. Check at home before putting it away that it's safe.
3. Before cooking/serving, confirm that it's safe.

So what happened for us to get three strikes? Well, first these fish sticks had come as part of an online order so we had not checked at the store. Second, the food was delivered in the middle of a hot summer day. I wasn't home and Jay was on a work call, but he zipped downstairs, brought the food in, and quickly put away all the perishables before rushing back to his meeting. He had not had time to review all ingredients as he performed the quick task. Third, on the day of the reaction, I had included my kids in dinner prep before the beach. I gave Thomas the job of putting their food on a cookie sheet and in the oven for me. Shea had chosen fish "sticks" and Thomas had picked fish "squares" as we called them. While similar, they hadn't selected the same dinner that night. I had not trained him to review ingredients since Jay and I usually did this. An area for improvement looking back because both kids were certainly old enough and capable of reviewing ingredient lists. It would have been good practice for them. I didn't think about any of this when I served my kids their dinner that evening.

There it was. Our three strikes.

Ok I thought. But she loves these fish sticks and we've bought them so many times before. How is there suddenly milk in them? Then we noticed. The type we typically bought was gluten-free and milk-free. This box was not. They looked nearly identical! We certainly couldn't fault the grocery store employee who mistakenly grabbed this box. One of us could have made the same mistake. I was so upset about how similar the boxes were that I later contacted the company and shared our story. I commended them for having great practices with transparent labeling and thanked them for making delicious products but I implored them to please make the packaging more distinct between their different products. I figured we weren't the first family to make this mistake and if they didn't address this I worried we might not be the last.

To be honest, as awful as it was to see the breakdown in our system, I appreciated knowing what had caused the reaction. At my dad's wedding we never really figured out exactly what happened. Knowledge is power and it helped to know so we could avoid that same mistake moving forward.

Shea was totally freaked out by this reaction though. She was anxious. At the time I didn't realize how much it affected her. She wasn't telling us all the thoughts she was having. Much of it wouldn't come out for nearly a year. Superstitions she called them, but really they were anxieties. For instance, she was nervous to eat dinner on Sundays (the day it happened) at 5:20 (the time it happened). She was afraid to wear the shorts she had worn that day. She was afraid to wear the bathing suit she had worn that day. She was afraid to sit in the chair she had been sitting in when we gave her the epi. The list went on once she started opening up about it. It took time but as she was able to verbalize these anxieties we were able to support her. We worked to replace her fears with safe experiences. Slow and steady.

I felt like we had handled the reaction in textbook fashion. We knew what caused it so it wouldn't happen again, and we saw our errors so we could learn and do better in the future. But all she processed was "Disaster." At my dad's wedding she had been much younger and wasn't as impacted emotionally. Back then she let us worry for her, but as she has grown up she has taken on far more of the worry than is good for someone her age. More than we realized.

She refused to eat fish sticks after that. I have to cook most nights. We don't get a lot of "easy nights." We never get to say "oh, let's just grab a pizza on the way home." Fish sticks were easy! Throw them on the pan, throw it in the oven, and boom dinner is ready. It was hard to lose an easy dinner option, especially because the correct fish sticks were still safe. Eventually she tried them again, but she had lost that loving feeling for them and I'm not sure when she'll get it back. I was pissed. Angry. Mad. So fed up with food allergies. I had never had such a strong, negative, emotional response about my kids' allergies. After it happened I shared a post about it, to remind friends to check ingredients and be aware of packaging that could lead to confusion. A friend reached out and said "Meg, if this can happen to *your* family then it can happen to anyone." Right. So what good did all my education and awareness work do? I hadn't prevented this from happening.

And then another blow. While still managing my anger following Shea's reaction we faced another reaction. It was Christmas Eve. Friends of ours kindly dropped off some sweet treats for our family which has been a tradition of theirs for years. There were two types of homemade treats, one safe and one not. Thomas was so excited to try something homemade! After asking, he picked one out and gobbled it up with a smile. Within a matter of minutes he said, "Mom, my throat feels funny." And he was flushed. Shoot. Maybe there had been cross-contact? Over the next few minutes he started to feel worse. I asked Jay to call our friends to see what the ingredients were. That's when we discovered it. In the excitement of checking out the goodies, a mistake had inadvertently been made and he had eaten the wrong treat. Jay stared at me as he repeated what he heard over the phone "Ok, so there's dairy in those." My stomach sank. I looked at Thomas and gently said, "Well honey, we know you ate some dairy by accident and that's why you're feeling sick. I'm so glad we have your epinephrine for moments like this. I'm going to go get it so we can help you feel better." He cried a little but nodded. He was scared. Jay handed me his Auvi-Q and I pressed it against his outer thigh while he sat on the couch. Then I rubbed the area for a few seconds and asked Jay to call 911. Within minutes Thomas said "Wow, I already feel better." Thank goodness. Not long after, paramedics arrived. They monitored him. He was doing well. They made an exception and allowed us to skip the ER based on three things. First, they made sure we had additional epinephrine on hand in case the reaction started back up. Second, COVID numbers in our local hospital had spiked. Third, it was Christmas Eve. We spent the rest of the night monitoring him and I woke up a few times throughout the night to make sure he was ok. Thankfully, he was fine. The epinephrine had done its job. Dr. Pistiner had taught us, "if it's not read-able it's not eat-able" and here we had broken another one of our own rules.

But, again, we had known what to do. Shea had a PTSD type response to Thomas's reaction. She was so worried about him. And yet, it was good for her to see the epinephrine worked. He was ok. Even with an accident like this, we were prepared. We have learned over and over again that properly managing our children's food allergies means we have to maintain a healthy balance of prevention and preparedness. Both are necessary.

Food allergies can be hard. They don't give you a day off. They don't care if it's a holiday or a special occasion. And we aren't perfect. Accidents happen.

The question is, will you know what to do?

Because that's what matters most.

A Journey Not a Destination

"Travel isn't always pretty. It isn't always comfortable. Sometimes it hurts, it even breaks your heart. But that's okay. The journey changes you; it should change you. It leaves marks on your memory, on your consciousness, on your heart, and on your body. You take something with you. Hopefully, you leave something good behind." ~Anthony Bourdain

When Shea was first diagnosed with a milk allergy I assured myself that as a former classroom teacher I was prepared to handle this. I told myself, "I've got this." Also, Jay is a smart guy so I knew he'd learn and we'd take it in stride. But as she got older, it got harder. It was a lot more challenging to keep her away from milk and dairy products than I had anticipated. I hadn't understood what it would be like to socialize with other little ones who could eat her allergen. I hadn't understood how tricky it would be at family gatherings when much of the food was unsafe and we would have to plan our own food. I hadn't understood the level of trust needed if I was going to leave her in someone else's care, and the preparation required between education and food planning.

When Thomas was diagnosed I was less "clueless," but still felt like we had it under control. Accidents could happen and if we were just more careful things would be ok. If we were just as careful as possible we could handle it.

But then Shea had the anaphylactic reaction at my dad's wedding. Just one bite of cake and the rug was pulled out from under me, from us. I was more scared, more confused, and felt more alone than ever before. Everything I thought I knew came into question. Everything I thought I trusted I now worried about. It felt like I had to start from scratch in learning how to be a food allergy mom. In time I became acutely aware of the gaps that existed between diagnosis and daily life management. These gaps are where most of the challenges existed. I wanted to identify many of these and work to fill them.

Isolation was a gap. Starting SAFE was a significant step in my journey. I went into it looking for connection and to feel less alone. Along with that I learned how to lead a support group, how to access available funding, and how to organize events, guest speakers, and member engagement activities. Sometimes it was really hard work and I would think, *what am I doing?!* But whenever I get positive feedback or I'm told something I did helped someone, I'm reminded it's worth it. So much has come from connecting with others. Realizing I wasn't alone and that other families knew the struggles I knew, helped. Meeting families who knew the fear I knew, but who also knew successes I hadn't yet known, helped. Meeting families who had ways of doing things I hadn't yet thought of, also helped. There was power in these connections that I'm forever grateful for.

Feeling like nobody else understood was a gap. When I decided to create my first training class I became even more excited about ways to help others. While SAFE has primarily been about supporting other caregivers and families with food allergies, the classes I will be teaching for Food Allergy Allies are primarily meant for those outside the food allergy community. I want to keep things as fun and interesting as possible, not scary and not fear based. There is a lot of fear already. In my experience most people are kind, thoughtful, and want to help, but we need to guide them. We need to answer their questions, or better yet, answer questions they don't even know to ask. I want to provide useful information that is research and experience based, not fear based.

Learning that school districts don't necessarily have the level of food allergy management you'd like to see was a gap. I had to learn a lot about school management plans and advocate for the food allergic community in my district. This was uncomfortable at first, but in time I found my voice. A voice that would help me again and again in the coming years. Knowing that my efforts mattered not only for my children but also for those coming up behind us gave me a sense of purpose that kept me from crying in a corner thinking we were alone. Don't get me wrong, there were days like that in the beginning.

By the time Shea had her second anaphylactic reaction things had changed. I wasn't as scared, sad, or lonely as I had been the first time. I was mad. I hated that this could happen to my child, to other children, to other people. It had been six years and I had learned so much. And yet, accidents happen. Real life gets messy and we cannot control everything that happens. The silver lining was knowing exactly what to do. I still get frustrated by food allergies. I still want a better way of life for food allergic individuals and their caregivers.

I hope the future holds options beyond avoidance.

Until then, we can look for beauty in the gaps. Like the wonderful people my family and I have met on this journey. My kids have met older kids with food allergies who they look up to and who they've been able to ask questions of. They've similarly been able to support kids younger than themselves and answer their questions. These relationships are gifts. Food allergic kids have to "grow up" faster than many of their peers and are often faced with their own mortality younger than their peers. They learn to speak up for themselves at an early age. This is a useful life skill to have. They learn to advocate for themselves and step out of their comfort zones before they may feel ready. This eventually becomes their norm and has great value in life. From a young age they watch and learn from what is modeled for them, like how to order at restaurants, how to handle shared food moments. They learn how to do things for themselves with increased confidence which even some adults struggle with. I often tell my kids, "Everyone is dealing with something and you can't usually tell by looking at them." Food allergies is one of their things, but there is so much more to them than that. We can find beauty hiding in the gaps from diagnosis to daily life.

We can also remain hopeful. Stay hopeful that your efforts will have a greater impact than you might realize. We don't always get to see the fruits of our labors. Lucky for me, my sister's children attend the same elementary school that my children did. You know what she told me? That food is no longer part of elementary school classroom parties. Wow. After all the years and difficulties and awkwardness and admittedly, tears, it may have actually helped move the needle for those coming behind my family. That makes me happy.

More than 20 brave individuals contributed to the Interview section of the book. They answered the questions for me, but ultimately, for you. If you know someone managing or living with food allergies, ask them these questions. They just might appreciate an opportunity to answer and share some of their own story.

- ◊ What's the best thing about having (or managing) a food allergy?
- ◊ What's the most challenging thing about having (or managing) a food allergy?
- ◊ What advice do you have for someone newly diagnosed (or managing) a food allergy?
- ◊ What advice do you have for someone who has never had (or managed) a food allergy?

For now, we stay vigilant and keep the emergency plans and epinephrine prescriptions up to date. We live life to the fullest. We celebrate good days and special occasions the best ways we know how and we learn from difficult days. We talk with others and figure out how to approach new things safely. We team up and push for better legislation and increased awareness. We visit with friends and family. We make memories. And we know, every day, we are not alone.

Food-Free Fun

Over the years we've tried to get creative with ways to have fun. What other families did for fun weren't always options for us and we didn't have a lot of extra money to pay for activities. I came to discover that we thrived when events and activities didn't have a focus on food. And I liked when they didn't cost much. Some of our family's best experiences have been when the playing field was level. When food was taken out of the equation and my kids were just like their friends. As I've mentioned previously, there is often an emphasis on food. Breaking bread together is important, but when you have restrictions you think about food differently. You know food has the potential to be divisive and exclusive and dangerous. When you really start to think about activities that aren't around meals or food use, there are so many options! So many fun activities just waiting for you. It can be easy to get caught up in what you can't do, what's not safe, what feels like you're excluded from, but you can intentionally focus on what you can do, what's fun, what's safe, and what puts a smile on your kids' faces. Then invite their friends to show them that fun can happen without food!

Here are a few of our family's favorites....

 Go for a hike: Usually a free option, this is a nice way to enjoy the great outdoors. An organization near us created Quests (like scavenger hunts), and Geocaching is another fun idea. Or you can always make your own!

 Snow Adventures: Everything looks different when covered in snow. Brighter and more inviting. Venture into the woods. An old fallen tree suddenly becomes something to play on. A holly bush they never noticed before suddenly becomes the perfect hideout. Leave the woods and go sledding. Make a snowman or an igloo, let your creativity run wild!

 Beach Fun: Swimming, making up games, body surfing, building towers with beach stones, building sand castles, burying each other in sand, jumping off rocks and swimming back to shore, having contests to see who can hold their breath the longest, using snorkel gear. The beach has tons of free options.

 Dance Parties: Crank up the tunes and open the dance floor! Invite friends and use a garage, driveway, deck, yard, even a room in your house with furniture pushed aside. Have water available so everyone stays hydrated!

Talent Shows: Talk with some friends and see who has a skill they want to share. Make a list and invite parents, neighbors, friends. Have someone emcee and introduce each act then sit back and enjoy the show! Microphones and lights are helpful but not necessary.

 Jump Rope: There are fun jump rope rhymes you can practice. Use a shorter rope for just yourself or get a good long one and have multiple people try jumping together. Coordinate your moves like choreography. Exercise, fun, laughter, all for free once you have the jump ropes.

 Gardening: Oh how I love this! What's your preference? Cut flower garden? Vegetable garden? Our family has had a vegetable garden for years. The kids help with selecting the items, planting, weeding, and then the real fun comes in harvesting, cleaning, and prepping what we grew to eat. Our favorites are lettuce, kale, spinach, green beans, and cucumbers. Automatic salad! Obviously only grow food that is safe for your family.

 Making music: The sky's the limit with this. What instruments do you and your friends play? Who likes to sing? Partner up and make it happen together... who knows, you might be starting a future famous band! Karaoke anyone?

Interviews

"Nothing we learn in this world is ever wasted."
~ Eleanor Roosevelt

My voice is loud in this book, but it is by no means the only voice in the landscape of those managing food allergies. Additionally, I wanted to provide space to learn from others, to hear their perspective, whether similar or different from my own. As you will see, the following individuals fit one of three categories – parent/caregiver, food allergic adult, or food allergic/celiac child. Each was asked the same four questions:

BEST THING

What's the best thing about having (or managing) a food allergy?

MOST CHALLENGING

What's the most challenging thing about having (or managing) a food allergy?

ADVICE FOR NEWLY DIAGNOSED

What advice do you have for someone newly diagnosed with (or managing) a food allergy?

ADVICE FOR NON FOOD ALLERGIC

What advice do you have for someone who has never had (or managed) a food allergy?

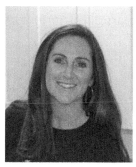

Meghan Neri

Stay-at-home mom, educator, consultant

Manages: milk, peanut, tree nuts

BEST THING

Best thing is becoming more connected to what we eat. You learn to read ingredients and when you simplify to more whole foods and fewer processed foods (because they can be confusing and risky) you often eat healthier. I have thanked my kids many times over the years for having food allergies because it has helped all of us eat healthier.

MOST CHALLENGING

Worst thing is fear and confusion. Fear of accidental exposure or ingestion. Confusion about how to handle tricky situations that usually involve other people. You don't want to seem "needy" or "pushy" but you want to keep your children safe. Social avoidance seems easy because it can eliminate some fear and confusion but that also comes with it's own issues.

ADVICE FOR NEWLY DIAGNOSED

Advice for others managing is that you are not alone. I remember the first time I met another allergy mom. I remember the first time we met a child as allergic to milk as Shea was. While current statistics show that 1 in 13 kids have food allergies, you don't always know who, and they may not have the same allergies. Finding a way to connect with others who understand has been such a helpful part of my journey.

ADVICE FOR NON FOOD ALLERGIC

Advice for those who don't manage is that for many people food means stress. It is helpful when we can take the focus off of food when possible, like with school parties or sports. Private functions are another thing. Since it's nearly impossible to meet the needs of all allergies or other dietary restrictions that might be connected to such a function, being clear and up front about the menu gives others a better opportunity to bring their own similar, safe substitutions.

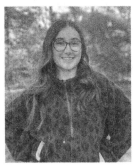

Shea Neri
9th grade
Allergy: milk

BEST THING

You're different. You have a story to tell. No matter what someone says, I have my story to tell. Everyone's food allergies are different which means their experiences are different. If I'm telling my friends something food related and someone asks "what are you talking about" I have my story to back it up.

MOST CHALLENGING

Anxiety and always worrying that something bad is going to happen. Also, hearing about bad things that have happened to other people. I feel bad for those people first and foremost.

ADVICE FOR NEWLY DIAGNOSED

Find what works for you. Everybody is different and that's something you need to accept. Accept who you are.

ADVICE FOR NON FOOD ALLERGIC

Try to be understanding and try not to make it awkward. Maybe ask "what do you like to eat" instead of "how can I make this safe for you," because half the time we don't know how to answer that and it's awkward.

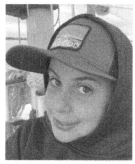

Thomas Neri

6th grade

Allergies: milk, peanut, tree nut

BEST THING

Being able to participate in things for people with food allergies, like the FARE Conference and SAFE activities.

MOST CHALLENGING

That you have to watch your friends eat food that you want to eat, but you know if you eat it you might not be here anymore.

ADVICE FOR NEWLY DIAGNOSED

Don't eat what you're allergic to. It'll ruin your day, your night, or your morning.

ADVICE FOR NON FOOD ALLERGIC

Food allergies aren't a joke. Even if someone hasn't had a reaction that doesn't mean they don't have the allergy.

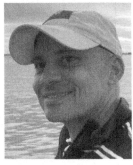

Jay Neri

Software Engineer

Manages: milk, peanut, tree nuts

BEST THING

Increased awareness of what goes into food and how food manufacturing works, as well as what we're actually putting into our bodies. Things might be safe but not healthy.

MOST CHALLENGING

The lack of freedom and relaxation/comfort from being able to go out to eat or have someone cook for you. There is fear – is this going to go well? Are the kids going to be happy with what they get, or disappointed?

ADVICE FOR NEWLY DIAGNOSED

Find support as soon as possible so you don't feel like you're alone. Find options for how to deal with certain situations from people who've been through it already.

ADVICE FOR NON FOOD ALLERGIC

Be as compassionate as possible. You only know what you know when you need to know it. It's a more complex problem than maybe it sounds on the surface. There is often an anxiety piece for the kids and even the adults that doesn't always seem logical. Like why someone might not want to eat something even though it's supposedly safe for them to eat.

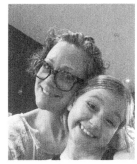

Jackie Scoon

Chef

Manages: egg, peanut, tree nut, sesame, dairy

BEST THING

I feel like I've become a champion for my family. Like this crazy cheerleader advocate. Being a woman in a kitchen I've had to be assertive. I was assertive in my work life but not my personal life before this. It was very hard for me in the beginning but I push and I push and I've been able to get things done, like hand sinks in our preschool.

MOST CHALLENGING

I have no control. I can't be with my kids 24/7 and when they're not with me I feel like I'm not in control, like I'm not managing the allergies. We've had to teach them that they are each in charge of themselves (when they're not with us).

ADVICE FOR NEWLY DIAGNOSED

Never let your guard down. Always read labels then reread them. It's a lot to manage but it's all going to be okay

ADVICE FOR NON FOOD ALLERGIC

Be respectful. If I say no, you may not feed my child, don't take it personally. Be understanding that I don't think your house is dirty. I don't think you're dirty, I don't even trust myself sometimes. Nobody looks at surfaces, like a stovetop or something, the way a food allergy parent does.

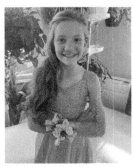

Ellie Mark

5th grade

Allergies: severe dairy

celiac disease

BEST THING

I would say the best part is getting special access to things like events for people with food allergies and getting to board planes first. It's also the best that I meet other kids with the same things going on.

MOST CHALLENGING

You can't have the same food other people have, or go to restaurants a lot. Sometimes you have to miss out on fun things because of allergies. Some kids would say EpiPens are the hardest part but they aren't the worst thing – they help. I have had to use so many EpiPens that it's not too bad.

ADVICE FOR NEWLY DIAGNOSED

I would give them the advice not to think of it as a bad thing. Think of it as something that makes you different and it could always be worse. Doctors are learning much more now about food allergies to make things better for people with allergies.

ADVICE FOR NON FOOD ALLERGIC

Please don't make fun of people with food allergies. Don't say "oh I LOVE cheese" or some allergen, when you talk to someone with an allergy. Does that make sense? Try to understand and listen to people who have had allergies for a long time.

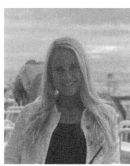

Ariel O'Shea

Teacher

Allergies: peanuts, tree nuts

BEST THING

That's tough. I don't know if there is a best thing. In hindsight if I look at it as a positive thing I can't eat nuts, and they have a lot of fat so I eat less of that. Also, you eat healthier foods and you learn to be more careful about what you put into your body. Last, having an allergy has put me at an advantage of understanding others who have food allergies. I have some students with food allergies, and when they find out I do too they don't feel so different. It's like, hey guys, I get it.

MOST CHALLENGING

Being out. Even at family parties and having to speak up and say hey I have an allergy. I was always a shy little kid and wasn't one to say I have an allergy, I can't eat certain things. It makes me feel a little embarrassed to be honest. I'd be one of the only ones who couldn't eat something or couldn't be in the same room as something that had nuts in it. It was challenging. The way my friends joked about it made me feel uncomfortable. They were kidding around but it hit a little bit of a nerve. I wished I could eat that Reese's peanut butter cup. I laugh about it and roll with the punches but it does hit a nerve.

ADVICE FOR NEWLY DIAGNOSED

Be very on top of it. Don't stop enjoying life, just be aware, be outspoken. It can be as simple as, "I have a nut allergy, what's in this food?" Be confident. It's more accepted now. Or, let someone know who will help speak up for you. I have a friend who does that for me and I just love her for it. It's not the end of the world to have food allergies. It can feel overwhelming but there's still a lot of things you can eat. I can eat plenty of natural foods, fruits and veggies.

ADVICE FOR NON FOOD ALLERGIC

You're blessed. Try to have some empathy for others who might have food allergies. It's hard because people have different allergies. Don't be afraid to ask them about it. Be open minded about it. Don't be like "that sucks for you". Ask questions, try to empathize.

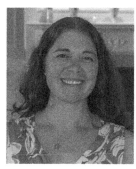

Lauren White

Stay-at-home mom

Manages: peanuts, tree nuts, eggs, dairy, wheat, soy, sesame

BEST THING

For my family the best part about managing food allergies was becoming more aware of what we were eating and the ingredients in all of our food. I also love all of the other food allergy families that I have been lucky to connect with!

MOST CHALLENGING

Missing out on social events. We have been managing food allergies for almost 15 years now, so it is much more rare that we would have to miss out on something because of food allergies. When my daughter was younger and we were less familiar with how to deal with certain situations there were many times when we just chose not to go to a social event rather than try to figure out a way to make it work. These were usually last minute things, like a group of preschoolers going to a last minute pizza party after school and I just couldn't get a safe pizza for my daughter in time, so we chose to skip it.

ADVICE FOR NEWLY DIAGNOSED

Reach out to other families who have been managing food allergies – I learned all the best tips from other moms! And give yourself some grace – this is hard and we are all doing our best.

ADVICE FOR NON FOOD ALLERGIC

Listen to the families who are managing food allergies, they know what will work best for their kids and that might be different from what you assume will be best. Also – be kind! Food allergies are very stressful and there is a huge learning curve for families. Sometimes we might not be as patient as we would like, but we are just trying to keep our kids safe.

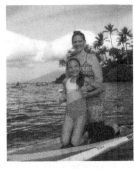

Ann Mark

Educational Consultant

Manages: severe dairy allergy, celiac disease

BEST THING

The community of people I've met. Also the support I've gotten and that I've been able to provide to other people. From doctors to others like Melissa Engel (the Lead Programming Developer of Teen Outreach with FARE) and organizations like FARE.

MOST CHALLENGING

Most challenging is the lack of inclusion of my child. Seeing her get left out of things. Seeing people try so hard to include her but actually being so exclusive. Almost like drawing attention to it. Watching her emotions of not being included. It's frustrating that we're not what's considered "acceptable" allergy mainstream like peanuts.

ADVICE FOR NEWLY DIAGNOSED

Find what's normal for your and your family. Find providers that work as a collaborative team with the parents. Find who works with you and what works for you. And as a parent, find support for yourself because you can't project your fear and anxiety onto your kids. Find a way to manage it outside your kids.

ADVICE FOR NON FOOD ALLERGIC

Listen to the people who have been there. Listen to those who manage them. Listen to the resources and providers. But don't give input back. You don't have a place to contribute here. Just be an ally. Allies are so important. Listen to why my kids have these needs and how you can be an ally.

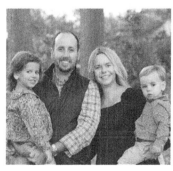

Leah Crowley

Finance manager

Manages: milk, eggs, peanuts, tree nuts, shellfish, sesame

BEST THING

All that I've learned about food and ingredients. Going into this I knew nothing about food allergies or reading a food label or anything like that. And the impact that certain ingredients can have on consumers.

MOST CHALLENGING

1) The preparation. Advanced prep before we go anywhere... meals, snacks, what type of food might be there, do we need to bring utensils? 2) When we aren't with her, the fear that she could consume something she's allergic to without us knowing or being able to help her

ADVICE FOR NEWLY DIAGNOSED

You're the advocate for your child. When you're eating with other people, with friends, with families, you need to educate them. They may think you're being too controlling or that you don't trust them but you need to protect your child and you know what they can or can't tolerate. People don't always know how to read labels the way we do.

ADVICE FOR NON FOOD ALLERGIC

Be patient if you're with someone who has food allergies. To the extent that you can, educate yourself about how severe food allergies can be. "She'll probably outgrow it," might be someone's way of trying to be positive, but it can be frustrating when you've heard from doctors over and over again that it's not a likely possibility.

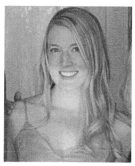

Jenna White

Pediatric Occupational Therapist

Allergy: sesame

BEST THING

Being a picky eater I can use it as an excuse when there's a food at a party that I wouldn't want to have anyway. Not be rude, but also not have to eat a food I'm not sure about.

MOST CHALLENGING

The anxiety about it. For a long time I would feel so nervous going out to eat if my girlfriends wanted to go out. I'd have to look up the restaurant, look at the menu, and try to figure it all out ahead of time. Anxious about not wanting people to be annoyed with me, but also with not wanting to go to the ER. Watching people go to restaurants and they get to eat anything they want and not have to worry about it.

ADVICE FOR NEWLY DIAGNOSED

Read every label because the majority of times my issues came from me eating something that I assumed didn't have my allergen without actually putting my eyes on the label and then having an anaphylactic reaction.

ADVICE FOR NON FOOD ALLERGIC

To understand the severity of it and not judge someone for not wanting to go somewhere or ordering something and asking people to double and triple check everything.

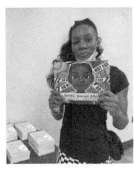

Meerah Mincy

Parent of a 4th grader

Manages: shellfish allergy

BEST THING

Like many things in life, managing food allergies is one of life's many lessons. The food allergy being the teacher and those with the diagnosis are the student. The student learns patience, advocacy and discipline all in which apply to daily life situations.

MOST CHALLENGING

Managing food allergies presents very challenging situations as a parent of a 10-year-old. In a society where children want to fit in and be cool, not being able to enjoy shellfish with friends is disheartening. Eating takeout food with the possibility of cross-contamination is unfortunate and creates a sense of fear and uncertainty that causes panic and hatred for the diagnosis.

ADVICE FOR NEWLY DIAGNOSED

To anyone newly diagnosed with a food allergy "chin up." You are not alone, you did nothing wrong. Do your research, ask questions, share your diagnosis if comfortable with loved ones. Advocate for self when in settings that may trigger your allergy.

ADVICE FOR NON FOOD ALLERGIC

For those who have never managed a food allergy, be kind. Be understanding. Do research if curious and do not judge. Food allergies can appear at any age.

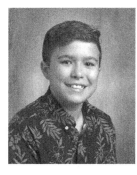

Colin Hood

6th grade

Allergies: dairy, egg, soy, beef, sesame, peanut, tree nut, coconut, lentil, chickpea, pea, legumes, millet, spelt (also off wheat, gluten, carrots, food dye for EOE)

BEST THING

Food allergies, unlike many other known diseases, can be avoided and you can live a normal life. You can still eat some other foods with care. I think my diet is healthier because I can't eat a lot of things that are fatty or unhealthy in different ways due to the allergens. It feels so much better when you get to eat a new food. It is such a bigger deal when you finally find a new thing that you can eat! I don't think people without food allergies have the same appreciation for new foods, or just eating in general. It has allowed me to connect to many people that I wouldn't have met otherwise... like through FARE. I have gotten to meet Senators and help pass laws to help change the future for other people with food allergies.

MOST CHALLENGING

The worst part is having to think about what you can and can't have at every meal and everywhere you go. Sometimes getting excluded from a birthday party or having to sit somewhere else when at an event where there is food. Having to be constantly aware of everything around you and what you are touching. For example, every time I go to a restaurant I have to give them an allergy card, wipe down all surfaces, and put in three extra steps more than someone without food allergies just to be able to maybe eat there. Even then I might have to eat food I brought from home. Having the actual allergic reaction is one of the worst times ever. They can be different each time, painful, throwing up, throat closing, hives, and maybe even die.

ADVICE FOR NEWLY DIAGNOSED

Allergies are avoidable. They suck, but they are avoidable. An epipen might seem scary, but it is probably the most life-saving thing for people with food allergies. You might not be able to have some foods that other people get to eat... and sometimes you won't be able to eat food at all... but you can still live the life you want. I have played on sports team, I have friends who support my food allergies and have learned to use the epi pen, you get to go on vacations and do mostly normal things. Food just isn't the focus. Don't be scared to try new foods if they are safe. I am nervous most of the time when I try a new food, but when I discover a food I can have it is GOOD! If you have a reaction, make sure you are around someone that knows how to use the epi pen. Don't get scared in a way that you are doing dumb stuff. Make the smart choices even though it is scary. Don't move a lot if you think you are having a reaction. An allergy is just like any other disease or disability. We don't have control over the disease, but we can control the situations... even how you manage the reactions.

ADVICE FOR NON FOOD ALLERGIC

People can die of food allergies. Take them seriously and don't just breeze over it when someone tells you they have one. Treat people with food allergies equally. We just want to feel normal. We are the same as you, we just might not be able to eat the same foods as you. Take into consideration how much harder the lives of food allergy people are... and also that they can die from this. People sometimes don't wash their hands, or say "I'll wash hands later" or not take a request about food or cleaning seriously. But to the food allergy person, these are life-saving things.

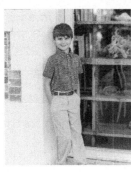

Cody Geise

5th Grade

Allergies: peanuts, eggs, dairy/milk, chicken, sesame, sunflower seed, wheat

BEST THING

It helps teach responsibility and how to manage school and other situations. You are much more aware of your surroundings. It makes you more aware of yourself and your health.

MOST CHALLENGING

Not being able to eat food that looks and smells good. A lot of the precautions are needed to be safe that drive you away from a normal life experience. That can be difficult

ADVICE FOR NEWLY DIAGNOSED

Always be aware of your food and surroundings. Talk to your doctor, ask questions and find other people who have food allergies and can help.

ADVICE FOR NON FOOD ALLERGIC

Feel lucky you are able to enjoy all food. Don't take that for granted. Try to be understanding of people with food allergies. They don't have that freedom.

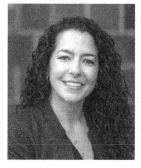

Christine (Chris) Creter

Learning strategist and facilitator for corporate adult education programs.

Allergies: peanut, tree nut, coconut, sesame, scallop

Manages: Dairy, egg, soy, beef, sesame, peanut, tree nut, coconut, lentil, chickpea, pea, legumes, millet, spelt (also off wheat, gluten, carrots, food dye for EOE)

BEST THING

The best part about having food allergies is the awareness it brings to eating. There is an appreciation for good, safe food that I don't think those without food allergies can relate to.

The best part of managing food allergies for my son is the community that I have found in other parents, organizations, etc. I don't know what I would have done without non-profits like FARE, or communities of people (in Facebook, support groups, etc.) that just "get it." I have felt empowered to help change laws at the state and federal level that will hopefully make things easier on people that come behind me with this life-changing diagnosis. I've been able to educate students and staff within our entire district, change policies to keep kids with food allergies safe, and raise awareness… thanks to the support and tools provided by the incredible network within the food allergy community.

MOST CHALLENGING

The anxiety is the worst part of having and managing food allergies. I am constantly thinking about the next meal, how many grocery stores we need to go to, what we might be running out of, and where we might find the food if it is out of stock again. The anxiety of being in seemingly "normal" social situations is amplified the minute food is involved. Exhausting hypervigilance... watching what everyone is eating, who is or is not washing their hands, what they are touching, where my son might come into contact with these foods, etc. Avoiding these situations isn't an option, otherwise I risk socially isolating my son. (It's always been important to send him the message that you can live a very full life, we just need to plan ahead and be careful.) But that doesn't erase the anxiety as a mom watching my son at a birthday party either be left out of activities, or included but with the fear of a reaction. Most other parents of kids that don't have food allergies, don't get the anxiety we carry. I have had many people say "don't worry, he'll be fine" or "you've got to let him learn to live with these food allergies" but they have no idea what that means in reality. Another "worst part" of food allergies are the lack of options available to us and the effort that goes into food. We can't just decide to go out to dinner if a soccer tournament goes long, or we bump into friends. We have to plan ahead for any possible food situation... and not just having food available, or knowing where we MIGHT be able to eat out... but also for keeping food hot, or cold, and the hygiene element (hands, utensils, plates, pots/pans, grills, surfaces, etc.). A baseball double header means kids eat food in between games... so I make sure to have tons of wipes and casually ask everyone to wipe their hands before playing ball (all without drawing too much unnecessary attention to my son.) I have been in situations when we didn't think we would be out long enough to span a meal, and been caught with nothing... desperately trying to find a safe bag of potato chips or whole fruit we can wash just to tide him over until we can get to food that is safe. As a mom, I first want my son safe. And I also want him included. Balancing these two things is the hardest thing I do on a daily basis.

ADVICE FOR NEWLY DIAGNOSED

Join a community, read everything you can (from reputable sources), crowd-source ideas for treatment AND food/recipes... but don't let anyone tell you their way is the only way. You will find what works best for your family, given your unique set of diagnosed allergies and how you manage them. For example, voluntary food labeling (may contain, made in a facility with, made on shared equipment...) is not regulated so different families have different tolerance levels for what they are willing or comfortable eating based on these labels. Whatever you have researched or whatever risk you are comfortable assuming based on these is up to you! Empower your child to manage their allergies as early as possible. Have them carry their own chef cards, ask questions, read labels, inquire at restaurants, gauge whether or not they feel safe at the restaurant based on the responses of the staff, practice using the trainer devices, and self-carry or self-administer as early as professionals say they are ready. Also know that IT GETS EASIER! It seemed completely overwhelming to me at first, but in time I realized I could manage this and still help my son have a fulfilling life. He has gone long stretches of time with no reactions at all. While it is important to stay vigilant in those times when you start to feel "safe," you can also celebrate the length of time you have gone without a reaction! And finally, you will make mistakes. I have accidentally fed my son an allergen resulting in a reaction. I have had to administer epinephrine and go to the hospital. While there are stretches of time with no reactions, that stretch will likely end. And you can't let it break you. You have the knowledge of the allergies and how to do your best to prevent them, and the tools to treat a reaction if it happens (always carry two epinephrine auto-injectors!), and don't beat yourself when/if a reaction happens.

ADVICE FOR NON FOOD ALLERGIC

First, I ask people without food allergies to imagine what it is like to be afraid you will die several times a day. If you can even grapple with the idea that you can legitimately be at risk of this several times a day, you might begin to understand the gravity of this hidden disease of food allergy. I know kids look "normal" and it might seem like people are going to extremes to avoid foods or asking you or your kids to wash their hands to avoid food protein cross-contact situations, but these small steps help reduce that risk of going into anaphylaxis or dying.

So my advice is to simply listen to the food allergic child or parent, and recognize that anything they are asking you to alter is because they are trying to increase their chances of staying alive. Please don't minimize the seriousness of food allergies and the vigilance needed to prevent contact with food proteins. At the same time, don't isolate people because of it either. Don't let your fear of having the food allergic kid around keep you from inviting them to a playdate or birthday party, or putting them in an isolating situation. Simply ask the parent or even the child what we can do to help keep them safe. This willingness to have the conversation alone will let us food allergy patients and caregivers know that you are taking it seriously, and we can work together to allow the kid as normal an experience as possible with some inclusive, agreed-upon, safety measures in place. It is likely easier than you might think!

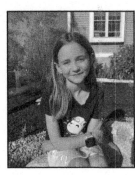

Ena Scoon

2nd Grade

Allergies: peanuts, tree nuts, eggs, dairy, sesame

BEST THING

I think during Halloween that we get to have the teal pumpkin and give out toys to kids not candy. It's so fun and you get to share. I love going to Amy's!

MOST CHALLENGING

When people change the ingredients. How you think something is safe and then it's not. Why would they do that? It's not easy for the parents because they have to look at every single ingredient. It's not needed. It takes up a lot of time.

ADVICE FOR NEWLY DIAGNOSED

If people pick on you, let it slide. You're unique in your own special way. It doesn't matter if they say you're different. It matters how you feel. You'll get used to it, I'll tell you that. It's ok if kids pick on you, because who cares about their opinion. Only your opinion matters.

ADVICE FOR NON FOOD ALLERGIC

Always tell your parents if your friend has an allergy. If they don't know, your friend could end up in the hospital. It's not every day you have a friend that has allergies. It's ok when someone has allergies.

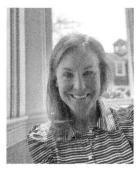

Muffy Antico

Active mom of 5

Has managed: tree nuts, dairy, sesame, egg, wheat, soy

BEST THING

The best thing about managing food allergies is that it actually makes me stop and look at what I'm giving my kids on a regular basis. What is it that we are putting in ourselves? Oddly enough, another blessing is that it gave me another thing to connect with my food allergy kids with. We stop and have one more thing we do together. They aren't fun but we are a team. The team aspect of it. This is one thing we can work on together. It helps keep me connected to their world.

MOST CHALLENGING

The most challenging thing truly is the emotional side of keeping my worries in check when we are out places. Managing the anxiety of my child and myself. Trusting a restaurant or a chef that they are doing what they said they would do. I can fix whatever food I want at home and control that environment but the hardest part is when we can't control the environment.

ADVICE FOR NEWLY DIAGNOSED

I'd say it's going to be ok. You can do this. It's not the end of the world, it's about making other choices that aren't mainstream. Look for the other choices, they are there. I wish someone had told me it would be ok.

ADVICE FOR NON FOOD ALLERGIC

For someone who's had no experience with food allergies everybody gets nutrition one way or another. Because someone is making choices that weren't familiar to you doesn't mean that they aren't doing well or not happy. Everybody has to do with they have to do. Don't judge. In my house we say "don't yuck someone's yum." What works for us may not work for you.

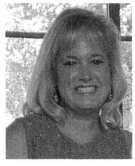

Denise Bunning

Mom, former teacher, support group leader

Manages: milk, tree nuts, shellfish, fish

BEST THING

Hmmm. Well, it's not like you wished for your children to have life-threatening food allergies or Eosinophilic Esophagitis... however... the experiences (good, bad, and ugly) have educated us as a family to be organized, self-sufficient, empathetic, and grateful.

MOST CHALLENGING

Worst things about managing food allergies are food challenges, having an anaphylactic reaction, being in the hospital and/or ICU! Scary stuff.

ADVICE FOR NEWLY DIAGNOSED

Advice for someone who is new to managing food allergies is to get a great pediatric or adult allergist, educate yourself and your family, join FARE and a local or online support group, and always have your medication with you.

ADVICE FOR NON FOOD ALLERGIC

Advice for someone who has never managed food allergies is that food allergies are a REAL disease that can end a life. Please treat people with kindness and respect. Just as you would any other disease or disability that you could see.

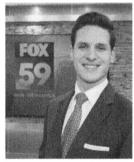

Tucker Antico

Broadcast Meteorologist

Allergy: tree nut

BEST THING

The best thing about having food allergies is that it keeps me healthier. When I'm out and people are offering dessert, even if it's someone who seems to know what they're dealing with when it comes to food allergies, I tend to be cautious. I tend to avoid desserts which has helped keep me healthier.

MOST CHALLENGING

The most challenging thing for me personally has changed over time. When I was little all the way up until about college, it was an anxious thing. Even eating food from people I trusted. It was harder in grade school and middle school when I didn't quite have independence to buy my own food. As an adult I buy my own food and choose my own restaurants so it hasn't been as big a deal for me. Now it's more about always being aware of my surroundings and situations. It's always kind of in the back of my mind, and I need to make sure I'm in control. I don't eat when I'm drinking, unless I'm certain. I never want to end up in a bad situation.

ADVICE FOR NEWLY DIAGNOSED

Advice for someone new to managing food allergies would be to always have your epi pen. There's a good chance you might never have to use it but it can be life or death for people, and until you have a reaction you don't know how it might be. Just because you had one reaction that wasn't anaphylaxis doesn't mean it'll be the same next time. Don't take unnecessary risks. Make sure people around you understand and make sure you are conformable with a situation if you're going to be eating. Maybe you're at someone's house and you don't feel totally comfortable but you don't want to be rude. It's best not to ever feel pressured into eating anything. Be ok with advocating for yourself, or doing it for your child if you're a parent.

ADVICE FOR NON FOOD ALLERGIC

When it comes to people who do not have allergies, I appreciate all the people in my life who take it seriously. Friends, girlfriends, or anyone I go out with know about my allergies. I just say hey, I have a nut allergy. If something happens I have my EpiPen or Auvi-Q, and I'll show them how to use it. I've never had anybody act like it's a joke. There have been times at restaurants with waiters and waitresses saying things like "I think you'll be ok with that," but this isn't an "I think" sort of thing. I want them to take it more seriously. In general, I have found people my age seem to know food allergies are serious. If they ask questions to learn more it shows me they respect it and take it seriously, which makes me feel more comfortable being around them. Peers are important. They will be my first responders if I need them.

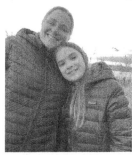

Greenie Morrissey

4th grader

Celiac Disease

BEST THING

The best thing about having celiac disease is Celiac Camp in Rhode Island. I'm glad I was diagnosed young so I won't be sick all of my life like some other people.

MOST CHALLENGING

The most challenging thing about having celiac disease is seeing other kids eating normal food that I can't eat.

ADVICE FOR NEWLY DIAGNOSED

Advice for someone new to managing celiac would be don't feel left out, a lot of people have celiac disease. Educate yourself about the disease so you know what you can and can't eat.

ADVICE FOR NON FOOD ALLERGIC

Advice for someone who has never managed celiac disease is try to understand how hard it is to deal with. And to take it seriously. Being glutened sucks!

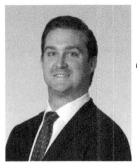

Paul Urbank

Sales Director

Allergy: all nuts

BEST THING

A huge benefit to having a food allergy is developing a great awareness and knowledge of the ingredients of the foods we consume. There is also a strong sense of community and support with others that have a food allergy.

MOST CHALLENGING

The most challenging thing for my allergy is how prevalent peanuts and nuts are. Although awareness has increased significantly over the years, I still feel peanuts and nuts are used a lot as cooking oil or healthy alternatives in meals and snacks. It is imperative to be aware of your surroundings and carefully read the ingredients if you are unfamiliar with the product.

ADVICE FOR NEWLY DIAGNOSED

Don't be afraid to ask questions. You need to be very diligent and ask about not only how the food is prepared but what ingredients are used.

ADVICE FOR NON FOOD ALLERGIC

Food allergies are more than just an inconvenience. It is important to learn about food allergies and understand the symptoms of an allergic reaction and how to recognize them.

Resources

FARE | Food Allergy Research & Education

www.FoodAllergy.org

AAFA | Asthma and Allergy Foundation of America

www.aafa.org

FAACT | Food Allergy & Anaphylaxis Connection Team

www.foodallergyawareness.org

SAFE | South Shore Allergy Family Educating

www.southshoreallergyfamilies.org

Allergy Eats | The Leading Guide to Allergy Friendly Restaurants Nationwide

www.allergyeats.com

Allergy Home & Living Confidently with Food Allergy Handbook

www.allergyhome.org

MA State School Guidelines for Managing Life-Threatening Allergies in Schools

www.johnstalkerinstitute.org/wp-content/uploads/2020/06/Mng-Allergies.pdf

CDC Voluntary Guidelines for Managing Food Allergies In Schools and Early Care and Education Programs

www.cdc.gov/healthyschools/foodallergies/

Equal Eats | Food Allergy Translation Cards in 50 Languages

www.equaleats.com

The Food Allergy Counselor | Your Allergy Psychosocial Resource Hub

www.foodallergycounselor.com

Food Allergy Stages Handouts | American Academy of Allergy Asthma & Immunology

www.aaaai.org/Tools-for-the-Public/Conditions-Library/Allergies/Food-Allergy-Stages-Handouts

Kyle Dine | A Trusted Educator with a Twist

www.kyledine.com

The Land Of Can | Inspiring Young People to Embrace a CAN Mindset

www.thelandofcan.com

About the Author

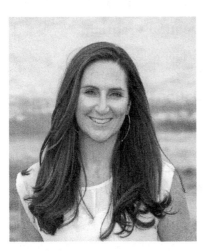

A food allergy mom for more than 14 years, Meghan Neri has lived the ups and downs of daily management. After facing challenges along the way, her number one goal became trying to make the journey easier for those coming behind her. A former school teacher, she knows the importance of education. In 2017 she co-founded a food allergy support group called SAFE (South Shore Allergy Families Educating), which is a FARE (Food Allergy Research & Education) recognized support group aimed at connecting caregivers and working to increase awareness and education in the community. More recently she founded an education and consulting business called Food Allergy Allies (foodallergyallies.com), with a mission to increase the safe inclusion of food allergic individuals through intentional education. When she isn't teaching or talking about food allergies you can find Meghan at the beach with friends and family. By the sea is her favorite place to be.

Made in the USA
Monee, IL
11 June 2023

35549724R00154